Medulloblastoma - Therapeutic Outcomes and Future Clinical Trials

Edited by Thomas J. FitzGerald

Published in London, United Kingdom

Medulloblastoma - Therapeutic Outcomes and Future Clinical Trials
http://dx.doi.org/10.5772/intechopen.1002105
Edited by Thomas J. FitzGerald

Contributors
Amir Azarhomayoun, David Harris, Eric Ko, Fran Laurie, Gavin Jones, Hebah Abudawaba, Jessica Yancey, John M. Buatti, Julia Hayden, Julie Trifone, Koren Smith, Linda Ding, Maryann Bishop-Jodoin, Maryann Bishop-Jodoin, Matthew Iandoli, Naheed Usmani, Nura El-Haj, Parisa Zafari, Paul Rava, Sandy Kessel, Stefanie Lowas, Thomas J. FitzGerald, Thomas W. Smith, Vinaya Rajahraman, Yansong Geng

First published in London, United Kingdom, 2025 by IntechOpen
IntechOpen is the global imprint of INTECHOPEN LIMITED, registered in England and Wales, registration number: 11086078, 167-169 Great Portland Street, London, W1W 5PF, United Kingdom

For EU product safety concerns: IN TECH d.o.o., Prolaz Marije Krucifikse Kozulić 3, 51000 Rijeka, Croatia, info@intechopen.com or visit our website at intechopen.com.

British Library Cataloguing-in-Publication Data
A catalogue record for this book is available from the British Library

Medulloblastoma - Therapeutic Outcomes and Future Clinical Trials
Edited by Thomas J. FitzGerald
p. cm.

This title is part of the Oncology Book Series, Volume 1
Series Editor: Thomas J. FitzGerald

Print ISBN 978-1-83769-622-2
Online ISBN 978-1-83769-621-5
eBook (PDF) ISBN 978-1-83769-623-9
ISSN 3049-8864

If disposing of this product, please recycle the paper responsibly.

IntechOpen Book Series

Oncology

Volume 1

Aims and Scope of the Series

The field of oncology has undergone extraordinary change and progress over the past several decades. Today, information is evolving at a rapid rate, with standards of management far different than standards of care applied during the training of most practicing oncologists. Oncology practitioners in all disciplines must remain current to optimize patient care. Basic and translational science remain critical in developing process improvements for patient care. The closer we understand the mechanism, the more we can improve targeted therapies and apply them to patient care. The pace of information is moving faster than at any previous time in history, and all oncology disciplines must remain current to provide excellent service to patients. The modern oncologist must be fluent in using big data and the volume of information generated in clinical trials. As we move closer to personalized patient care based on genomics and molecular biomarkers, the modern oncologist has to be nimble in assessing all available information and how this would be applied to each patient, balanced by the clinical status and medical co-morbidities of each patient. Targeted therapies can bring new and different sequelae, and oncology teams need to remain fluent in managing the consequences of therapy and primary management. In this book series, we will present how modern care has progressed in multiple disease areas and how modern oncology teams need to adapt in order to manage the cancer patients of today successfully. Surgery, radiation therapy, and medical oncology are practiced today with the support of exceptional modern technology, and in this series, we will review how these improvements are applied to each disease site to maintain excellence in patient care.

Meet the Series and Volume Editor

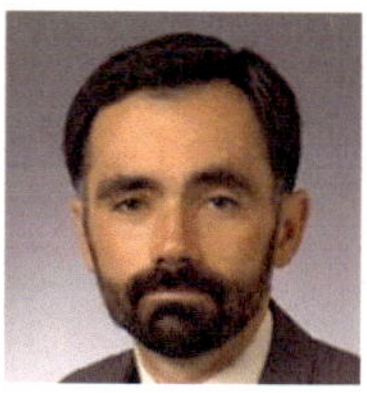

Dr. FitzGerald is the professor and chair of the Department of Radiation Oncology at UMass Chan Medical School in the USA. He serves as one of the principal investigators of the Imaging and Radiation Oncology Core (IROC) service for the National Cancer Institute clinical trials program and is directly involved in the quality assurance of clinical trials in the National Clinical Trials Network (NCTN). Dr. Fitzgerald manages NCTN clinical trials with a real-time pre-therapy review of imaging and radiation therapy treatment objects to ensure the care plan complies with study objectives and the patient stage has been assigned to the correct study. His basic science interest is in hematopoietic stem cell biology and cellular adhesion molecules as they pertain to therapeutic resistance and mitigation of injury from therapy.

Contents

Preface

It is a privilege to present this textbook on medulloblastoma. This is a complex disease with a significant history of management. Early pioneers in surgery recognized that the disease had access to the fluid pathways within the central nervous system, and the therapy pattern needed to align with the natural history of the disease and pattern of spread. While surgery could address the obstructive component of the disease, surgical removal did not generate a durable outcome and radiation therapy with limited orthovoltage techniques was applied to address the pattern of failure. Although improved tumor control was achieved on occasion, radiation therapy brought sequelae to the patient, which led to permanent change and limited the quality of life of the cancer survivor. As processes for diagnosis, imaging, radiation therapy and chemotherapy matured, strategies for care and the approach to the patient improved as both technology and treatment delivery programs became more sophisticated. Today, the disease is characterized by molecular biomarkers and treatment can be titrated and augmented based on risk factors defined by pathology, imaging, and molecular expression products. Radiation therapy has become more sophisticated, and particle therapy with protons is increasingly important in improving patient outcomes.

In this book, we present both the history and process improvements associated with all aspects of managing this disease, as well as future insight into management.

Thomas J. FitzGerald MD
Professor/Chair,
Department of Radiation Oncology,
UMassMemorial HealthCare,
UMass Chan Medical School,
Worcester, MA, USA

Professor,
Departments of Pediatrics, Radiology, and Obstetrics/Gynecology,
UMassMemorial HealthCare,
UMass Chan Medical School,
Worcester, MA, USA

Principle Investigator,
Imaging and Radiation Oncology Core (IROC)/Quality Assurance
Review Center (QARC),
National Cancer Institute Clinical Trials Network (NCTN),
Lincoln, RI, USA

Chapter 1

Introductory Chapter: Medulloblastoma – Past, Present, and Future

Thomas J. FitzGerald

1. Introduction

Although medulloblastoma is an uncommon disease, it remains a common oncology disease in the pediatric central nervous system. The disease retains signatures of historical and modern oncology disease management. From the early moments of surgery, chemotherapy, and radiation therapy, current treatment reflects the significant process improvements in all disciplines, including imaging radiomics and biomarker-associated pathomics which are now directly associated with process improvements in modern patient care. It is important that we understand how therapy was applied in the past to appreciate the steps taken to improve patient outcomes.

2. History and modern care

The history and current management of patients with medulloblastoma represents the challenges and consequences of cancer care as well as the promise of future developments for therapy. It was recognized by Cushing that, despite the removal of visible disease in the fourth ventricle, the disease had a propensity to migrate through central fluid pathways within the central nervous system which would uniformly recur and lend to a guided prognosis. Surgery would alleviate symptoms generated by obstruction of the fourth ventricle, however, the amelioration of symptoms was all too often temporary, and disease would recur despite the best and optimal surgical efforts. Recognizing the limitations of surgery noted by the pattern of failure within fluid pathways of the central nervous system, visionaries including Paterson and Farr, developed a care plan with orthovoltage radiation therapy that could apply radiation treatment to tissues that could not be approached with surgery. The introduction of radiation therapy provided patients a therapeutic option with tumor control which could be durable. However, cancer therapy during this generation had limitations driven in large part by the consequence imposed by therapy on developing normal tissue as well as limitations of technology and treatment delivery systems. As the disease largely affects the pediatric population and tissues at risk involve large body volume segments, therapy plans have been challenging for decades due to acute and late effects of management. Tissues including developing central nervous tissue, bone, and endocrine tissue are directly affected by therapy and exit dose from the spine indirectly affect cardiac, pulmonary, bowel, hepatic, and gastrointestinal parenchyma. Although the disease would respond to radiation therapy, disease

IntechOpen

control requires radiation doses that would impose injury to tissues of both rapid and limited self-renewal potential. Therefore, patients surviving the disease would require management of the sequelae of therapy for a lifetime and endure the frailties imposed by cancer treatment. The introduction of chemotherapy to this disease was to address the need for improved disease control and potentially limit the sequelae of radiation management by using titrated doses of radiation to both primary and secondary target volumes. Chemotherapy can impose additional sequelae to normal tissue; therefore, providers of care post therapy need to address multiple issues moving forward which can be overlooked as patients transition from pediatric to adult care.

Management processes have significantly improved and hopefully, in time, the process improvements will promote improved outcomes relative to both tumor control and normal tissue tolerance. Surgical and anesthesia techniques have significantly improved, and surgical talent can secure excellent and safe surgical outcomes. Imaging tools including modern magnetic resonance imaging sequences have optimized our understanding of disease location and tumor spread which have been further enhanced by tools in radiomics and artificial intelligence. Radiation oncologists are becoming more clever in target volume definition and dose painting that have permitted further exclusion of critical normal tissue from therapy to further improve normal tissue outcome. Intensity modulation and applied modulation of proton therapy have permitted exclusion and dose gradients across the cochlea and key visual pathways to limit injuries imposed by both chemotherapy and radiation therapy. The vertebral bodies can now be excluded from the target volume, recognizing their relationship to the spinal cord and fluid pathways. Cardiac and pulmonary volumes can now be titrated by limiting exit dose from the spinal fields to these critical volumes. Therefore, step by step, radiation oncology is moving the field forward by limiting the dose to normal tissue. Eventually, we will learn to subsegment volumes at risk in the central nervous system and learn to dose paint within the central nervous tissue and deliver less dose to the tissue of intermediate risk of tumor recurrence. Clinical trials and careful assessment of outcome imaging will help us develop artificial intelligence tools to move these ideas to enterprise function.

Perhaps the most important advance in this disease is the evolution of molecular profiling and the association of biomarkers to outcomes. Clinical trials without biomarker knowledge have failed to demonstrate noninferior outcomes to radiation dose titration, however, we currently recognize favorable outcomes associated with the WNT biomarker, therefore, protocols can now be developed and executed revisiting therapy titration in favorable patients. Eventually, therapies can be developed to biomarkers which may further improve outcomes and limit sequelae to management. It is remarkable how far this field has come in the past decade. Drs. Cushing, Paterson, Farr, and all caregivers of the past would be pleased with both current care and the potential for continued improvements in the future [1–6].

Author details

Thomas J. FitzGerald
University of Massachusetts Chan Medical School, Worcester, MA, United States

*Address all correspondence to: tj.fitzgerald@umassmemorial.org

References

[1] Cushing H. Experiences with the cerebellar medulloblastomas: A critical review. Acta Pathologica et Microbiologica Scandinavica. 1930; **7**(1-2):1-86. DOI: 10.1111/j.1600-0463.1930.tb06503.x

[2] Paterson E, Farr RF. Cerebellar medulloblastoma: Treatment by irradiation of the whole central nervous system. Acta Radiologica. 1953;**39**(4):323-336. DOI: 10.3109/00016925309136718

[3] Jenkin RD. Medulloblastoma in childhood: Radiation therapy. Canadian Medical Association Journal. 1969;**100**(2):51-53

[4] Seidel C, Heider S, Hau P, Glasow A, Dietzsch S, Kortmann RD. Radiotherapy in medulloblastoma—Evolution of treatment, current concepts and future perspectives. Cancers (Basel). 2021;**13**(23):5945. DOI: 10.3390/cancers13235945

[5] Michalski JM, Janss AJ, Vezina LG, et al. Children's oncology group phase III trial of reduced-dose and reduced-volume radiotherapy with chemotherapy for newly diagnosed average-risk medulloblastoma. Journal of Clinical Oncology. 2021;**39**(24):2685-2697. DOI: 10.1200/JCO.20.02730

[6] Kahalley LS, Paterson R, Douglas Ris M, et al. Superior intellectual outcomes after proton radiotherapy compared with photon radiotherapy for pediatric medulloblastoma. Journal of Clinical Oncology. 2020;**38**(5):454-461. DOI: 10.1200/JCO.19.01706

Chapter 2

Medulloblastoma Diagnosis and Treatment

Parisa Zafari and Amir Azarhomayoun

Abstract

Medulloblastoma is the most common malignant brain tumor in children. About 16–20% of all primary brain tumors in children are medulloblastoma, and it accounts for about 40% of all cerebellar tumors in childhood. The incidence of medulloblastoma peaked in those aged 9 years and younger. Some of the most common clinical symptoms of medulloblastoma are headache, vomiting, vertigo, and ataxia. Additional manifestations that may occur include lethargy, irritability, motor or cranial nerve impairment, gaze-palsy, sphincter disorders, and back pain in those with spinal metastases. Imaging tests can help determine the location and size of the brain tumor. A computerized tomography (CT) scan or magnetic resonance imaging (MRI) may be done immediately. It is uncommon to do a biopsy, but it may be recommended if the imaging studies are not typical of medulloblastoma. The treatment for medulloblastoma depends on several factors, including clinical conditions of the patient and the size and location of the tumor. Treatment methods for medulloblastoma usually include surgery followed by radiotherapy, chemotherapy, or both. Treatment for medulloblastoma focuses on removing as much of the tumor as safely possible and relieving intracranial pressure. This three-part approach, surgery, radiotherapy, and chemotherapy, can increase the survival of patients by up to 75%.

Keywords: posterior fossa tumor, brain tumors, medulloblastoma, surgery, chemotherapy, craniospinal irradiation

1. Introduction

Medulloblastomas are embryonal tumors of the posterior fossa. They are the most common malignant brain tumors in pediatric patients. First described by Cushing and Bailey in 1925, these tumors derive from discrete neuronal lineages based on molecularly defined subgroups. Children and teenagers under the age of 16 are primarily involved. It can rarely occur in adults. Medulloblastoma in adults is usually diagnosed between the ages of 20 and 44.

Medulloblastomas account for approximately 20% of brain tumors in children and 1% of primary central nervous system in adults [1]. Medulloblastoma exhibits a bimodal distribution in children. Children age 4–9 years old had the highest incidence at 44%, followed by adolescents (10–16 years old) at 23%, and only a 12% incidence in infants/toddlers (0–3 years old). There is an overall male gender predilection with

IntechOpen

a male-to-female ratio that differs between molecular subgroups. Medulloblastoma affected males 1.5 times more than females [1].

There is no clear etiology for medulloblastoma. An association between medulloblastoma and viral infections, for example, early John Cunningham (JC) viral infections or human cytomegalovirus (CMV) infections in childhood, has been reported. The majority of medulloblastomas occur as sporadic cases. However, hereditary conditions have been associated with medulloblastoma, including (1) Gorlin syndrome, (2) blue rubber-bleb nevus syndrome, (3) Turcot syndrome, (4) Rubinstein–Taybi syndrome, and (5) Li-Fraumeni syndrome.

The five histologic subtypes of medulloblastoma include:

(1) Classic MB (2) desmoplastic-nodular (D/N) MB, (3) large-cell anaplastic (LC/A) MB, (4) melanotic MB, and (5) Medullomyoblastoma [1].

The classic types account for approximately 70% of medulloblastomas. They have a high invasive tendency and possess occasional neuroblastic differentiation. Desmoplastic variants are less aggressive than classic ones and account for 15% of medulloblastomas. Large-cell anaplastic medulloblastomas constitute approximately 10% of medulloblastoma, are typically located in the cerebellar vermis, and are highly aggressive. This type of MB has high mitotic and apoptotic activity and large areas of necrosis. The prognosis is poor and survival time is short after diagnosis. The last two variants are rare and comprise 5% of medulloblastomas [1]. The most recent WHO classification of central nervous system tumors has divided medulloblastoma into four molecular subgroups: Wingless-activated (WNT), sonic hedgehog-activated (SHH), Group 3 and Group 4. Each subgroup has distinguished molecular, demographic, and clinical characteristics. The WNT medulloblastoma is the rarest subgroup, accounting for 10% of all medulloblastomas, and is the subgroup with the best prognosis. The SHH subgroup accounts for 30% of all medulloblastomas and is characterized by aberration in the SHH signaling pathway. Group 3 tumors account for 25% of all medulloblastoma cases and this subgroup has the poorest prognosis. Group 4 tumors account for 35% of all medulloblastomas; this subgroup is the most common. These tumors have an intermediate prognosis, similar to the SHH subgroups (see Appendix A) [2].

2. Clinical presentation

Patients with medulloblastoma can present with variable manifestations. Clinical Symptoms often progress over several weeks to months, and it is not uncommon for patients to have an extended symptomatic period before initial diagnosis. The clinical manifestation of medulloblastoma is generally nonspecific; it presents with symptoms of a rapidly growing posterior fossa tumor [3].

Medulloblastoma symptoms can vary depending on several factors, including a person's age, the size of the tumor, the anatomic location of the tumor, the presence of disseminated disease, and the presence of hydrocephalus. The most common presentation concerns raised intracranial pressure, including headache, vomiting, and lethargy. The younger, nonverbal patient presents with behavioral change. Symptoms in younger children include listlessness, irritability, and vomiting. The complaint of older children and adults is headache, especially upon awakening in the morning. Vomiting without nausea is common in the morning since being recumbent increases intracranial pressure [4].

Often, symptoms such as vomiting cause the patient to undergo a workup of the gastrointestinal tract for a long time prior to consideration of the CNS. Double vision may be developed by stretching of the 6th nerve caused by hydrocephalus. The sixth cranial nerve can be compressed at the petroclival ligament, resulting in diplopia and lateral gaze palsy caused by hydrocephalus. More commonly, visual disturbances result from papilledema; however, they also may originate from cranial nerve palsy (most commonly CN IV or VI). Papilledema may be present in as many as 90% of patients. The fourth cranial nerve is usually compressed by direct tumor extension into the cerebral aqueduct. Fourth cranial nerve dysfunction causes the greatest difficulty when eyes are rotated medially and depressed (i.e., going downstairs).

Examination of the extraocular muscles may detect nystagmus, which can be related to a lesion of the cerebellar vermis. Although this sign is nonspecific since Medulloblastoma is most commonly located midline, unilateral dysmetria is less common in the cerebral signs than either truncal ataxia or a wide-based gait. Recent symptoms are easily observable on tandem gait. In children, the tumor most commonly involves the cerebellar vermis and causes gait ataxia more readily than unilateral symptoms [4].

Desmoplastic medulloblastoma is more common in adults. This type of tumor usually arises in the cerebellar hemisphere, and signs of ipsilateral cerebellar dysfunction in the arm or the leg are more common. Torticollis and head tilt can be a manifestation of accessory nerve or trochlear nerve palsy caused by direct tumor compression. Also, head tilt and neck stiffness, caused by meningeal irritation, are complications of tonsillar herniation below the foramen magnum. Spreading of medulloblastoma to the spinal cord may cause the following symptoms: Back pain, inability to control the bowel and bladder, difficulty in gait, and severe weakness from tumor compression of the spinal cord or nerve roots (e. g., radiculopathy) [4].

3. Diagnosis

Medulloblastoma (MB) remains a challenging entity due to its aggressive nature, particularly when affecting pediatric populations. The diagnosis and subsequent classification of MB are pivotal in determining appropriate treatment strategies and predicting patient outcomes. The intricate diagnostic process involves a series of essential steps that collectively contribute to a comprehensive understanding of the tumor.

The clinical evaluation of a patient suspected of having MB is crucial in establishing a baseline for further investigations. The clinical presentation of medulloblastoma is generally nonspecific and is similar to that of other posterior fossa tumors. Symptoms such as persistent headaches, unexplained nausea, vomiting, and neurological deficits often prompt medical attention, leading to a detailed assessment of the individual's medical history and presenting complaints. This initial stage sets the foundation for the subsequent diagnostic modalities and treatment decisions [5].

Imaging studies, including MRI and CT scans, play a central role in the visualization and characterization of MB. These imaging modalities not only help locate the tumor but also provide essential information regarding its size, extent of invasion, and involvement of critical structures.

Because of the heterogeneous nature of MB, it has heterogenous features on MRI. The tumor can demonstrate variable T1 and T2 intensities and different enhancement patterns. It may have calcification, hemorrhagic area, and cyst formation (**Figure 1**). MRI features and tumor location can predict MB subgroups. Magnetic resonance spectroscopy (MRS) and diffusion-weighted imaging (DWI) with apparent diffusion coefficient (ADC) maps provide new prospects to correlate imaging findings

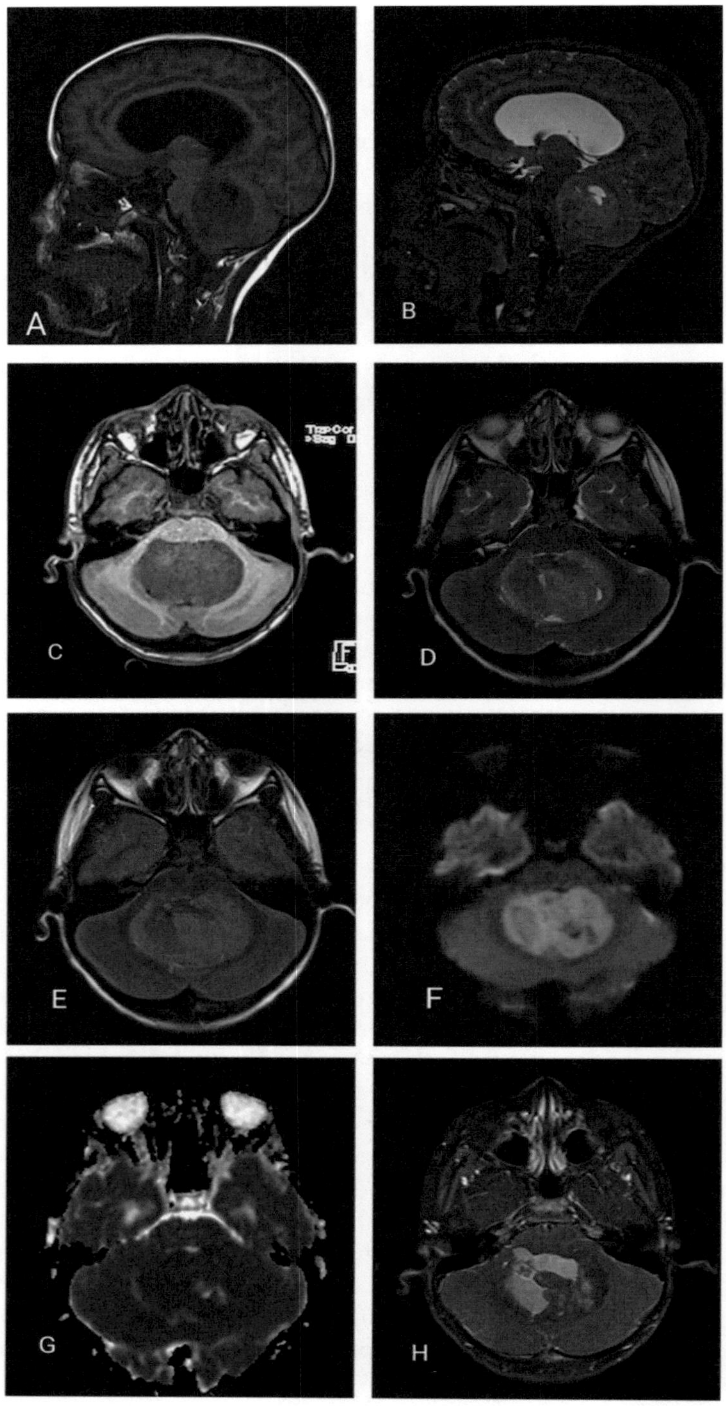

Figure 1.
A: Brain MRI T1 sagittal. B: T2 sagittal. C: T1 axial. D: T2 axial. E: FLAIR axial. F: DWI axial. G: ADC axial. H: T1 axial with contrast. MRI reveals the midline cerebellar mass, filling the fourth ventricle and compressing the brainstem and cerebellum. The tumor has a low signal on the T1 sequence compared with the surrounding normal cerebellum, mild hyperintensity on T2, heterogeneous enhancement, cystic/necrotic component, and diffusion restriction, manifested by high B1000 and low ADC value, indicating high tumor cellularity. The finding suggest medulloblastoma.

to medulloblastoma subtypes. The lowest and highest ADC values were observed in classic medulloblastomas and LC/A medulloblastomas, respectively [6, 7]. Tumor location was also found to be correlated with molecular subtypes. MRI features and tumor location can predict MB subgroups toward the cerebellar peduncle/cerebellopontine angle cistern originating from the lower rhombic lip. SHH subgroup had cerebellar hemisphere localization, and Group 3 and Group 4 originated from the vermis. Group 4 are characteristically nonenhancing tumors in the midline/fourth ventricle site, and this characteristic differentiates it from group 3 [8].

Leptomeningeal dissemination diagnosis is essential. Failure to detect leptomeningeal dissemination is one of the main reasons for treatment failure.

A whole-axis MRI with contrast or/and CSF cytology should be performed to detect leptomeningeal dissemination (**Figure 2**). Whole-axis MRI is often done preoperatively to evaluate metastatic disease. If preoperative whole-axis MRI was not performed, it is recommended to be performed more than 2 weeks after surgery [9]. CSF cytology test is the golden standard for the detection of leptomeningeal dissemination. CSF can be collected intra-operatively or through Lumbar puncture 2–4 weeks after surgery [10]. When MRI and CSF cytology results are in accordance, the diagnosis is more accurate, but these results are frequently not in accordance [11, 12]. Advances in high-resolution mass spectrometry (MS) techniques and CSF proteomics have enabled the identification of small amounts of cancer cells in CSF, although its clinical usage remains to be validated [13].

Histological analysis, achieved through examining a tissue biopsy sample, remains the cornerstone in definitively diagnosing MB. The microscopic evaluation of tissue sections enables pathologists to identify the distinct cellular features characteristic of MB, including high mitotic activity and a propensity for rapid growth. This histopathological confirmation is essential for initiating appropriate treatment protocols tailored to the specific tumor subtype [14].

Advancements in molecular testing have significantly enhanced our understanding of MB biology by allowing for the classification of tumors into distinct genetic subgroups. These subgroups, including the WNT-activated, SHH-activated, Group 3, and Group 4 subtypes, exhibit unique genetic alterations that influence disease behavior, treatment response, and overall prognosis. Molecular profiling has revolutionized the field of neuro-oncology by guiding personalized therapeutic interventions based on the tumor's molecular characteristics [15].

In conclusion, the complex diagnostic pathway for MB necessitates a multidisciplinary approach encompassing clinical, radiological, histological, and molecular assessments. By integrating these diverse modalities, healthcare providers can achieve a comprehensive understanding of tumor biology, guide personalized treatment strategies, and optimize patient outcomes in managing this formidable pediatric brain malignancy.

4. Prognosis of MB

MB, a highly aggressive brain tumor primarily affecting the pediatric population, presents a complex set of challenges in terms of prognosis and treatment outcomes. Progresses in demonstrative imaging, pathology, and molecular biology coupled with advancements in neurosurgical approaches, radiotherapeutic strategies, and systemic treatments over the last two decades have significantly improved survival results for MB [16]. Notwithstanding these advancements, the 10-year mortality rate of MB is 34.6% in children [16]. Traditionally, MB patients are classified into standard-risk and

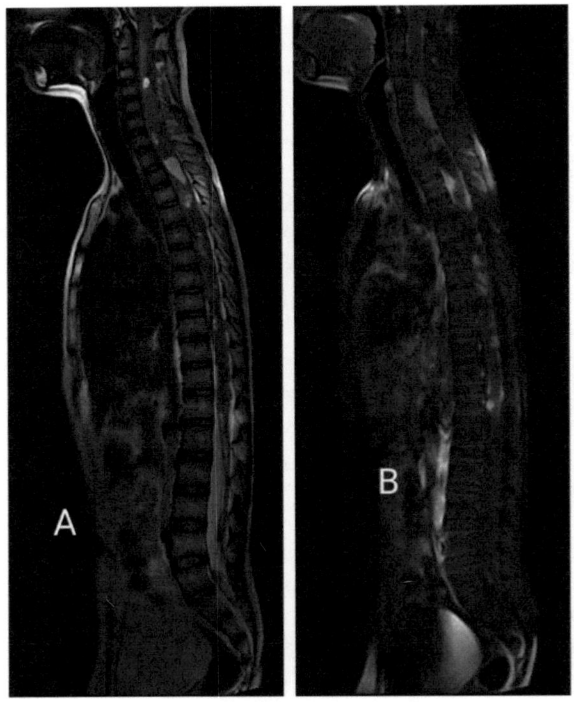

Figure 2.
A: Spine MRI T2. B: MRI T1 with contrast, fat sat (fat saturation). Diffusely bulky spinal cord, with shows extensive heterogeous enhancement. Multiple surface and nodular enhancing lesions in the spinal cord. These represent metastatic involvement of medulloblastoma.

high-risk groups based on clinical presentation, extent of residual disease after definitive surgery, histopathological group of the tumor, and biological or molecular characteristics of tumor cells [17, 18]. The 5-year survival rate of standard-risk patients aged ≥3 years old with current treatment is more than 70%. High-risk patients aged ≥3 years have a 5-year event-free survival (EFS) rate of around 70% for patients with metastatic BM treated with intensified chemotherapy regimens. Children beneath 3 years of age have a 5-year progression-free survival (PFS) rate of 30–90%, depending on tumor histology in this age group [17, 18].

The large cell/undifferentiated and classical subtypes have a poor prognosis, whereas the extensive nodular and desmoplastic/nodular MB have a better prognosis [17, 18].

The wingless/integral (WNT) subgroup has a good prognosis, the sonic hedgehog (SHH) subgroup and group 4 have an intermediate prognosis, while subgroup 3 has a poor prognosis [17, 18]. A recent meta-analysis suggests that the histologic characteristics of MB, molecular subgroups of MB, GTR, and radiotherapy are the most important prognostic factors associated with survival in patients with MB [19]. Epigenetic modifications, including DNA methylation patterns and chromatin remodeling, have emerged as critical determinants of MB prognosis. Specific epigenetic signatures within tumor cells have been associated with distinct molecular subgroups and survival outcomes. Epigenetic profiling provides a deeper understanding of the underlying molecular mechanisms driving tumor progression and may serve as a prognostic biomarker for risk stratification and treatment selection [20].

The immune system's role in mediating antitumor responses and shaping disease prognosis is a rapidly evolving area of research in MB. Immune checkpoint inhibitors, adoptive T-cell therapy, and other immunotherapeutic strategies have shown promise in harnessing the host immune response to target MB cells. The immunosuppressive nature of the tumor microenvironment, characterized by regulatory T cells and myeloid-derived suppressor cells, poses challenges for effective immune activation. Novel immunotherapies aimed at modulating the immune response hold the potential for improving prognosis and long-term outcomes in MB patients [21].

The treatment of MB, which typically includes surgery, radiation therapy, and chemotherapy, can lead to significant treatment-related adverse events affecting the patient's quality of life and long-term prognosis. Neurocognitive deficits, endocrine dysfunction, and secondary malignancies are among the potential complications associated with standard treatment protocols [22].

In conclusion, the prognosis of MB is influenced by a complex interplay of clinical, molecular, and environmental factors. A comprehensive understanding of the prognostic markers is essential for tailored treatment planning, prognostic assessments, and the continuous advancement of therapeutic strategies in managing this aggressive pediatric brain tumor.

5. Treatment

Treatment of medulloblastoma requires coordinated care by a neurosurgeon, neuro-oncologist, radiation oncologist, neuroradiologist, and neuropathologist. The current standard of care involves maximal safe surgical resection followed by risk-adapted craniospinal irradiation (for noninfant patients) and adjuvant chemotherapy. The goals of surgical management of medulloblastoma include maximal safe resection, obtaining tissue diagnosis, relieving mass effect, and treating symptomatic hydrocephalus. The extent of resection required has been closely studied, and residual tumor >1.5 cm^2 has been associated with worse overall survival and progression-free survival [23, 24].

5.1 Management of hydrocephalus

Hydrocephalus is a ubiquitous presenting feature in children with medulloblastoma. Hydrocephalus is common, occurring in 71–90% of children with posterior fossa tumors. Hydrocephalus after tumor resection occurs in 10–36% of cases, with a worldwide average of 30%. At times, it may require emergent intervention with external ventricular drainage (EVD) placement.

More commonly, patients will be symptomatic but not presenting in extremis and can be managed preoperatively with a short course of high-dose dexamethasone to treat peritumoral edema and with placement of an EVD at the time of surgical resection of the tumor. Although many patients require (cerebrospinal fluid) CSF diversion at the time of surgery, treatment with a ventriculoperitoneal shunt (VPS) or endoscopic third ventriculostomy (ETV) prior to tumor resection is not recommended because approximately 25% of patients require permanent CSF diversion. The risk of hydrocephalus requiring permanent CSF diversion in children with medulloblastoma may be higher in younger patients, patients with larger tumors, patients with metastatic disease, and patients with more severe or longstanding hydrocephalus. Patients with WNT subgroup tumors may also be at lower risk of requiring permanent CSF diversion [23, 24].

5.2 Surgery for medulloblastoma

Surgical resection is complete under general intravenous and endotracheal anesthesia. Patients are generally prone with the head fixed in a 3- or 4-pin cranial fixation device and the neck slightly flexed. In infants, the head may be positioned on a horseshoe headrest, taking care of pad-dependent areas and avoiding eye pressure. Care must be taken to avoid kinking the endotracheal tube with the neck flexed. This can be avoided by using a nasal endotracheal intubation technique or selecting an endotracheal tube less susceptible to kinking. Communication and coordination with the neurasthenia team is critical. First, a midline posterior fossa exposure is completed, exposing at minimum from the inion to C2. Dissection is undertaken in the midline avascular plane, and the cervical musculature is dissected from the occiput, bifid spinous process, and lamina of C2 in a subperiosteal fashion. Great care is taken in exposing C1, and a C1 laminectomy may be required, depending on the caudal extent of the tumor and the degree of acquired tonsillar herniation (Video 1, B2n.ir/g22558). Meticulous hemostasis should be achieved before opening the dura in a Y-or V-shaped fashion (**Figure 3**). Bleeding

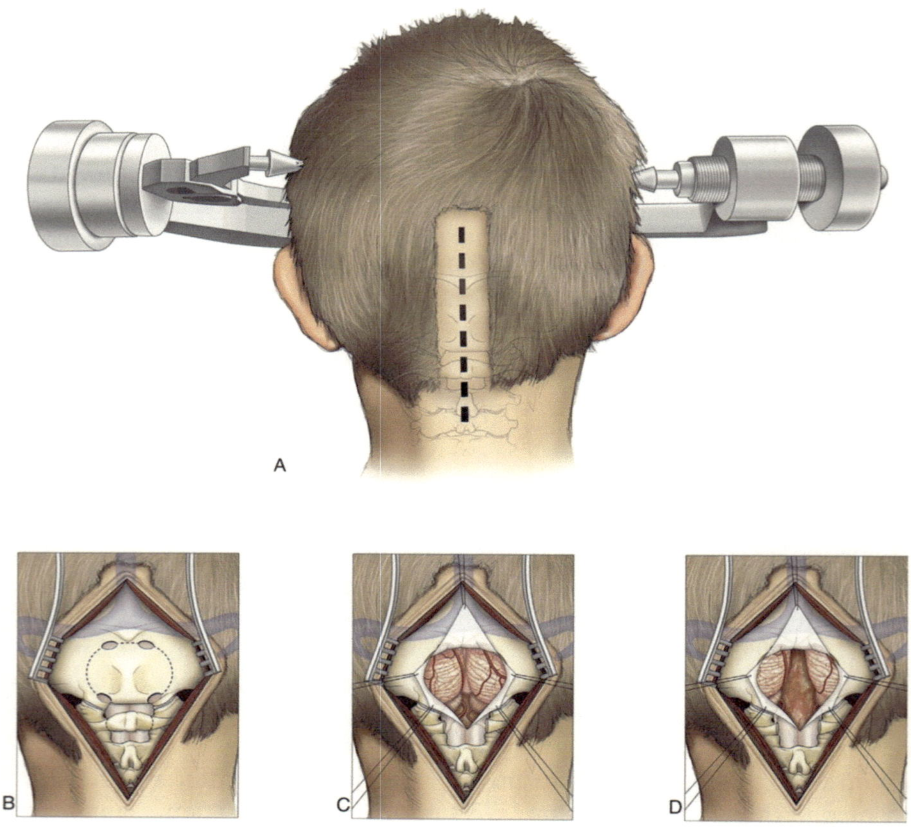

Figure 3.
(Schematic image) posterior fossa craniotomy and tumor exposure. A midine skin incision is made extending from just above the inion to the level of the spinous process of C2 (A). Bilateral burr holes are made and a craniotomy is performed incorporating the posterior rim of the foramen magnum (B). The dura is opened using a Y-shaped incision and the inferior cerebellum and brainstem are exposed. Care has to be taken to protect the posterior inferior cerebellar arteries (C). The dorsal surface of the tumor is exposed by divisionof the distal portion of the vermis (D). Posterior fossa and brainstem after tumor resection.

from the occipital sinus can be managed with Hemoclips (Teleflex Incorporated), which often can be removed at the end of the surgical procedure, thereby avoiding artifacts on postoperative MRI. A midline cerebellar vermian or inferior telovelar tonsillar approach can be used for midline tumors. In telovelar approach, the fourth ventricle is entered through the cerebellomedullary fissure, which is the virtual space between the medulla oblongata's posterior aspect and the tonsils' anterior surface.

The medullotonsillar space of the cerebellomedullary fissure and the uvulotonsillar space are sharply dissected to release the tonsils from the uvula and the medulla oblongata bilaterally. The telachoroidea is incised from the foramen of the magendie and then followed laterally to the foramen of the Luschka on both sides [24, 25]. This natural corridor provides access to the fourth ventricle without splitting the cerebellar vermis. A second advantage of this approach is the excellent view of the lateral recess of the ventricle and the exposure of the foramen of Luschka. The fourth ventricle is entered by splitting of the cerebellar vermis in the transvermian route. In this approach, the inferior vermis of the cerebellum is incised, and then the two halves of the vermis are retracted in opposite lateral directions. The inferior vermis is split on the suboccipital surface. The incision extends a variable distance through the uvula, pyramid, tuber, and folium of the vermis, depending on the location and size of the lesion. The following steps are in order: Retracting the two halves of the lower vermis laterally, then opening the telachoroidea and then inferior medullary velum, exposing the full length of the floor from the aqueduct to the obex. Total excision with minimal complications is the goal of the surgical tratment of the patients [24, 25].

Compared to the telovelar approach, it might offer a slightly better angle to reach the rostral part of the fourth ventricle. However, the transvermian approach is possibly associated with a higher rate of neurological complications [24, 25].

Both these routes may be useful for lesions that originate from the vermis. Identification of the floor of the fourth ventricle and brainstem is of critical importance in medulloblastoma surgery (**Figures 4** and 5).

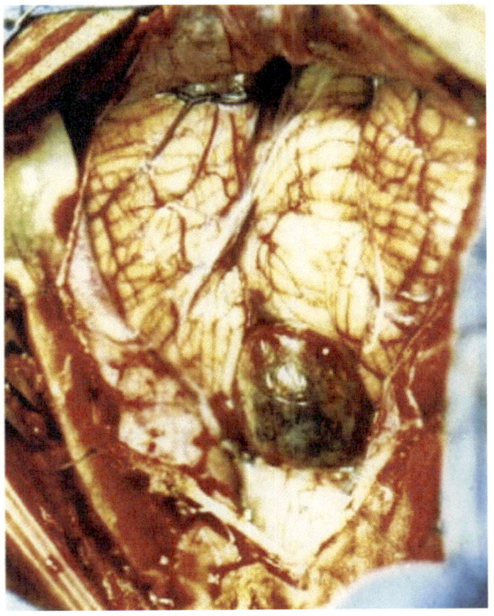

Figure 4.
Operative appearance of medulloblastoma prior to removal. Tumor is seen emanating from the fourth ventricle and displacing the cerebellar tonsils upward.

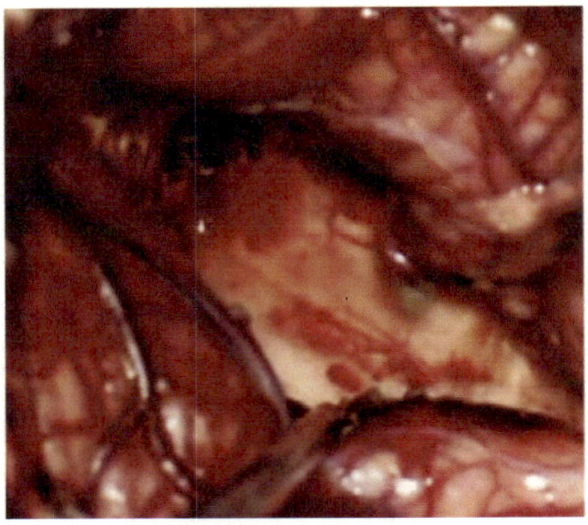

Figure 5.
At the completion of tumor resection, the floor of the fourth venticle is visualized.

It is useful to place a cotton patty at the ventral aspect of the tumor covering the floor of the fourth ventricle, as a marker to avoid extending the tumor resection to the brainstem. The margins of the tumor are dissected with a microsurgical technique to expose the interface between the tumor and the cerebellum. Samples of the tumor are taken for pathology review and diagnosis, and the tumor is internally debulked with suction and with a cavitation ultrasonic surgical aspirator. After the surgical resection, the cotton patty placed at the beginning of the resection, protecting the underlying fourth ventricle, should again be identified. The resection cavity is then inspected for any residual tumor before removal of the cotton patty. It is noteworthy that intraoperative neuromonitoring can be used to identify key structures. Continuous monitoring of the corticospinal and corticobulbar tract can be performed by recording motor-evoked potentials from limb muscles and facial muscles. Sensory pathways can be evaluated using somatosensory evoked potentials. Lateral/hemispheric tumors require a cordectomy through the overlying cerebellar cortex. Subsequently, tumor dissection, internal debulking, exposure of brain-tumor interface, and inspection for residual tumor will follow a course similar to that described for midline tumors. After tumor resection, meticulous hemostasis must be achieved with hemostatic agents, careful use of bipolar cautery, warm saline irrigation, and gentle tamponade with thrombin-soaked cotton balls. The dura is closed in a watertight fashion, using duraplasty when necessary. The bone is then replaced, and the cervical paraspinous musculature is reapproximated in the midline in a multilayered fashion. If an external ventricular drain (EVD) is required prior to tumor resection, a separate smaller incision can be made for placement of an occipital EVD. Cerebrospinal fluid (CSF) diversion with an EVD in the perioperative period is useful in managing hydrocephalus, ensuring appropriate wound healing, and avoiding the occurrence of a pseudomeningocele. The EVD can often be weaned over several days to a week postoperatively. In patients where permanent CSF diversion will be needed, it is prudent to avoid delay in placing the shunt to allow the patient to proceed with adjuvant therapy [24, 25].

5.3 Recurrence

MB recurrence occurs in approximately 30% of patients and is associated with poor prognosis. It is considered a serious complication. There is a wide range of therapeutic options, such as re-irradiation, surgery, chemotherapy, and targeted therapies.

Younger patients (more commonly, patients younger than 5 years) have a higher recurrence rate, and the role of histology is unclear. One of the negative prognostic factors is the detection of MYC amplification, which affects both the development of recurrence and time to death after relapse. The presence of metastatic dissemination at diagnosis had no effect on survival after relapse. Gross total resection and the absence of a residual or < 1.5 cm^2 residual tumor showed a lower recurrence rate. The molecular analysis revealed that the patients within the SHH subgroup and those with DN/MBEN histology have a better prognosis. On the contrary, non-DN/MBEN (desmoplastic, extensive nodularity) or subtotal resection (STR) within the SHH subgroup were considered poor prognostic factors. Group 3 usually presented with a disseminated relapse pattern and was characterized by MYC amplification, and Group 4 demonstrated local relapse and a moderate prognosis [26].

5.4 Complications of MB surgery

Surgical resection plays a central role in the management of MB, aiming to achieve maximal tumor removal while preserving neurological function. Despite advancements in surgical techniques and perioperative care, MB surgery is associated with potential complications that can impact postoperative outcomes and patient recovery. This section explores the common complications of MB surgery, their management strategies, and their implications on patient morbidity and long-term outcomes.

5.4.1 Surgical site infections

Surgical site infection is one of the most frequently encountered complications following MB surgery. Postoperative infections can arise from various factors, including prolonged operative times and CSF leakage. Prompt recognition and appropriate management of surgical site infections are critical to prevent further complications such as meningitis or abscess formation [27].

5.4.2 CSF leakage (pseudomeningocele)

CSF leak is a common complication observed after posterior fossa surgeries, including MB resections. Inadequate dural closure and inadequate closure of muscle layer, fascia, and hydrocephalus can lead to CSF leakage. Early detection and meticulous repair of the leak are essential to prevent the development of meningitis [28].

5.4.3 Hydrocephalus

The development of hydrocephalus following MB surgery is attributed to obstructed CSF flow or impaired resorption pathways. Postoperative hydrocephalus can manifest acutely or chronically and may necessitate the placement of a ventriculoperitoneal shunt for CSF diversion. Regular monitoring and prompt intervention are crucial in managing hydrocephalus-related complications effectively [29].

5.4.4 Cerebellar mutism syndrome

Cerebellar mutism syndrome (CMS) is a rare but debilitating complication observed in children undergoing posterior fossa surgery, including MB resections. CMS is characterized by a transient loss of speech and language function, often accompanied by emotional lability, motor deficits, and cognitive impairments. Rehabilitation and multidisciplinary support are essential in managing CMS and optimizing the patient's recovery and quality of life postoperatively [30].

5.4.5 Neurological deficits

Despite efforts to preserve neurological function during MB surgery, the procedure can result in new or exacerbated neurological deficits. Motor weakness, gait disturbances, sensory abnormalities, and cranial nerve palsies are among the potential neurological complications that may arise due to surgical manipulation or injury to adjacent vascular structures. Rehabilitation and neurorehabilitation programs are vital in facilitating recovery and function restoration in patients with postoperative neurological deficits [31].

In conclusion, understanding the potential complications associated with MB surgery is essential for healthcare providers caring for these patients. Early recognition, prompt intervention, and comprehensive postoperative management are key elements in mitigating complications, optimizing patient outcomes, and ensuring a successful recovery following surgical resection of MB.

5.5 Radiation therapy

Radiation has long been recognized to have an important role in the treatment of medulloblastoma, both to delay or prevent recurrence and to control metastatic disease. Work over several decades led to the adoption of a regimen of 35–36 Gy to the neuraxis and a boost to 54–55.8 Gy to the posterior fossa. It was shown that such a strategy led to consistent improvements in survival, the focus shifted to studying dose-reduction strategies for lower-risk patients to limit late toxicities. Currently, radiation protocols are tailored based on patient age and risk of relapse.

5.5.1 Risk-adapted therapy

Risk stratification: Patients older than 3 years old and have a tumor size<1.5 cm^2 after surgery are classified as the average-risk group. The presence of >1.5 cm^2 of tumor after resection and large cell anaplastic histology are considered a high-risk group. The recent molecular subgrouping of medulloblastoma will undoubtedly affect future risk-adapted treatment protocols [32, 33].

The low-risk group with a survival higher than 90% includes patients with non-metastatic WNT MB or non-metastatic Group 4 MB with genetic events such as loss of chromosome 11 or gain of chromosome 17 comprises patients with non-metastatic SHH MB with tumors without a TP53 mutation or MYCN amplification. Those with non-metastatic and non-MYC Group 3 MB are classified as the standard-risk group (survival of 75–90%). Patients with a metastatic noninfant, TP53 wild-type–type and MYC–amplified non-mastatic SHH MB and metastatic Group 4 MB are considered as high-risk and have a survival rate of 50–75%. The very high-risk group is considered as patients with SHH MB harboring TP53 mutations, or Group 3 MB with metastasis and has a survival rate of less than 50%. The patients with WNT and Group 4 may benefit from dose-reduced radiation with stable intellectual outcomes [32, 33].

For children older than 3 years old, postoperative radiation is performed as a standard of care. Average-risk patients may receive 23.4 Gy CSI and a higher boost of 55.8 Gy to the tumor bed, usually combined with weekly doses of cytostatic drugs as radiosensitizer 30 days after surgery. At the same time, those classified as high-risk patients are treated with 36 Gy CSI and an additional boost to 54 Gy to the tumor bed or posterior fossa and focal sites of metastases. The adverse sequelae, most deleterious in the youngest patients (<3 years), precludes using the approaches above in infants and young children. Therefore, in children younger than age 3 years, attempts are made to omit or delay radiation therapy or limit the use of focal radiation only. Because radiation dose-reduction studies have shown unfavorable outcomes with high relapse rates, primary chemotherapy followed by delayed radiation therapy is commonly employed for infants. Other groups defer irradiation to the time of first recurrence or after patients reach age 3 years or beyond [32, 33].

Alternative radiation technologies: Recently, the role of proton beam radiotherapy in treating medulloblastoma has been explored. With proton beam radiotherapy, the area targeted for radiation can be focused much more precisely, allowing the same dose of radiation to be administered with less effect of radiation to surrounding tissue. Proton beam radiotherapy also limits radiation to the spinal vertebral bodies, reducing late effects of scoliosis and short stature and exposure of the heart, lungs, and gastrointestinal tract. Additionally, if lower doses of radiation can be applied to critical areas of neurogenesis in the developing brain, a neurocognitive benefit to proton radiation may exist [32, 33].

5.5.2 Side effects of radiation therapy

Both short-term side effects and late toxicities limit radiation therapy for medulloblastoma. Short-term side effects include hair loss, fatigue, nausea, and vomiting, which can complicate or limit the successful completion of therapy. Late toxicities have become more apparent as long-term survival rates have drastically improved in recent decades. These late side effects include neurocognitive effects, neuropathy, endocrine abnormalities, growth retardation, scoliosis, hearing loss, cardiac toxicity, cerebrovascular disease, and secondary cancer. Neurocognitive effects are present in the majority of patients treated with CSI for medulloblastoma and include a severe reduction in their quality of life. Shorter attention span, slower processing, and memory disturbances contribute to a decline in executive ability and lower educational attainment. The main factor predictive of poor neurocognitive outcome is the young age at the time of diagnosis and treatment for medulloblastoma. Endocrine effects may include growth hormone deficiency, hypothyroidism, and early-onset puberty. Secondary malignancies are of significant concern as childhood medulloblastoma survivors live longer. These tumors include meningioma, malignant glioma, osteosarcoma, and myelodysplastic syndromes. However, alopecia and radiation necrosis are more common with proton radiation [32, 33].

5.6 Chemotherapy

Whereas historical treatment of medulloblastoma consisted of surgical resection followed by radiotherapy, multiagent cytotoxic chemotherapy regimens have evolved as a key adjunct therapy since 1970. Current chemotherapy regimens are risk-adapted, with differing strategies for average-risk children, high-risk children, and infants who undergo radiation-sparing protocols. Cytostatic drugs must pass the blood–brain barrier, and common chemotherapeutic agents are cisplatin, vincristine, cyclophosphamide, and lomustine.

Average risk: The current standard of care for classically defined average-risk children (age 3–18 years without metastasis and at least NTR) involves surgical resection followed by radiotherapy. Patients subsequently receive four to nine cycles of vincristine, cisplatin, and either lomustine (CCNU) or cyclophosphamide. These regimens result in 5-year overall survival rates of approximately 80% [32, 33].

5.6.1 High-risk children

Treatment of high-risk children harboring metastatic disease or significant residual tumors is less standardized, and most contemporary regimens used in recent clinical trials have resulted in 5-year survival rate of 50–70%. CSI plus tumor bed or posterior fossa boost combined with four to nine cycles of chemotherapy using combinations of is applied for high-risk patients. Conflicting data exist in trials comparing preradiation versus postradiation chemotherapy. Using a chemotherapy regimen consisting of three cycles of cisplatin and etoposide followed by seven cycles of vincristine and cyclophosphamide, Tarbell and associates investigated whether outcomes differed between high-risk patients when undergoing this regimen before or after radiation and found no statistically significant difference in overall survival (OS) (5-year OS of 73.1 and 76.1%, respectively). Intraventricular methotrexate has also been assessed as an adjunct to radiotherapy and cytotoxic chemotherapy for high-risk patients and resulted in 74% 5-year OS in patients 4 years of age or older with metastatic disease [32, 33].

5.6.2 Infants and young children

Because of the unacceptable toxicity of CSI on the developing brain, treatment of infants and young children with medulloblastoma typically employs chemotherapy-only approaches, with CSI reserved for use in progressive disease if the child has reached an acceptable age [32, 33].

The recognition of lower-risk infant groups based on histological subtype (DN) or molecular subtype (ish-II) has complicated the determination of ideal treatment strategies. However, it holds promise to find treatments that improve outcomes and reduce treatment-related toxicity. One approach has been to treat patients with high-dose chemotherapy combined with intrathecal methotrexate, resulting in the 5-year OS of 93% for patients with complete resection and no metastasis, 56% for patients with residual tumor but no metastasis, and 38% for patients with metastatic disease [32, 33].

5.6.3 Adverse effects of chemotherapy

Chemotherapy is associated with a variety of adverse effects, including acute events during treatment and chronic effects. Myelosuppression is extremely common, with grade 3 or 4 hematologic toxicity reported in nearly all patients, and can be a dose-limiting complication. Other acute side effects include fatigue, nausea, vomiting, anorexia, infection, and weight loss. Rarer side effects include nephrotoxicity, hepatotoxicity, cardiomyopathy, pulmonary fibrosis, and gastrointestinal toxicity. Ototoxicity resulting in sensorineural hearing loss is associated with cisplatin chemotherapy, requiring frequent monitoring and potential dose reduction. Treatment with multiagent chemotherapy may also have indirect consequences on long-term quality of life in medulloblastoma survivors [32, 33].

5.7 Novel therapies

Advances in understanding the molecular pathways that drive medulloblastoma tumorigenesis and the development of agents that block these pathways are paving the way toward targeted therapy for medulloblastoma. Inhibitors of the SHH signaling pathway, such as vismodegib or sonidegib, which target smoothened, have been trialed in SHH tumors. However, because of the importance of SHH signaling to skeletal development, SHH inhibition is restricted to mature patients skeletally. Additionally, the specific molecular alteration resulting in SHH pathway activation is important because patients with alteration downstream of smoothened (SUFU mutation or GLI2 amplification) are unlikely to respond to this therapy. The ongoing SJMB12 trial is incorporating vismodegib into maintenance chemotherapy in skeletally mature SHH subgroup patients. Other molecularly informed therapies have shown promise in preclinical trials, with some treatments, such as phosphoinositide 3- Kinase/mammalian target of rapamycin (PI3K/mTOR) pathway inhibitors, advancing to clinical trials. Various forms of immunotherapy have proved efficacious in preclinical models, and early-phase clinical trials are underway. Some studies have shown that simultaneous treatment with vaccination (such as with dendritic cells loaded autologous lymphocyte transfer) and chemotherapy improved antigen-specific T-cell activity. One of the successful approaches to treating several types of cancer is anti-HER2 chimeric antigen receptor T-cell (CAR T) therapy, and the HER2 receptor is also known to be overexpressed in medolloblastoma. Furthermore, a study titled Immunotherapy for Medulloblastoma in 2020, which was conducted by Kabir TF et al., showed that CAR T-cells could clear MB implanted in the posterior fossa in mice without any significant toxicity [33].

6. Conclusion

Medulloblastoma is the most frequent pediatric malignant CNS tumor. A multidisciplinary team that best diagnoses and manages medulloblastoma includes a pediatrician, neurologist, neurosurgeon, oncologist, radiation therapist, and specialty-trained nurses. Cerebellar symptoms are one of the first symptoms that the majority of children with medulloblastoma present to the primary provider. Once diagnosed, the treatment modalities for medulloblastoma combine surgical resection with chemotherapy and radiation. Recent molecular advances drive clinical trials and the development of novel therapies. However, there are still questions about how to best stratify treatment based on molecular findings and how best to combine targeted therapies with more traditional therapeutic mainstay. Progress and future trials will provide insight into these questions and ideally lead to better prediction of outcomes and decreased long-term deficits.

Acknowledgements

I am grateful to my colleague, Dr. Amir Azarhomayoun for his cooperation in preparing this paper.

Conflict of interest

The authors declare no conflict of interest.

Acronyms and abbreviations

MB	medulloblastoma
MRI	magnetic resonance imaging
CT	computed tomography
CSI	craniospinal irradiation
EVD	external ventricular drainage
ETV	endoscopic third ventriculostomy
CSF	cerebrospinal fluid
WNT	wingless
SHH	sonic hedgehog
D/N	desmoplastic-nodular
LC/A	large-cell anaplastic
TP53	tumor protein P 53

Appendix A

Medulloblastoma has been recognized to be a collection of distinct diseases, namely, the four molecular subgroups of medulloblastoma: Wingless (WNT), Sonic hedgehog (SHH), Group 3, and Group 4. Beyond the differences in underlying molecular biology, these subgroups have characteristic developmental origins, clinical manifestation, radiographic appearances, histopathologic correlates, and prognoses. Thus, molecular subgrouping of medulloblastoma informs all aspects of clinical practice, from counseling patients and their families to selecting appropriate treatment protocols to the long-term follow-up of medulloblastoma patients. These subtypes have important clinical correlates that will inform patient care and clinical trial design in the future. WNT Medulloblastoma is the rarest molecular subgroup, accounting for 10% of cases, but is associated with the best clinical outcomes with over 95% 5-year survival rates in pediatric patients. These tumors arise in children 4 years of age and older through early adulthood and occur with equal frequencies in males and females. WNT tumors usually have a classic morphology; however, 3% have LC/A histology. Nuclear localization of B-catenin is a hallmark of this subgroup. Metastases are present at diagnosis in 5–10% of patients, and the association of metastasis with prognosis in this subgroup is not well understood. Although recurrence is rare in this subgroup, both local and distant metastatic patterns of recurrence have been described. WNT tumors are driven by aberrant upregulation of the canonical WNT signaling pathway, which normally plays an important role in embryonic development. WNT pathway activation leads to cytoplasmic B- catenin accumulation and eventual translocation to the nucleus, where it activates transcription factors (T-cell factor/lymphoid enhancer factor-1) and induction of gene expression of downstream targets, including c-Myc (MYC) and cyclin D1 (CCND1). WNT pathway activation results in cellular responses, including cell proliferation and migration. Interestingly, the blood–brain barrier appears to be disrupted in WNT tumors, a unique characteristic compared to other subgroups, and this has been proposed as a mechanism for these tumors often appearing hemorrhagic at the time of surgical resection and being more responsive to standard-of-care treatment with cytotoxic chemotherapy.

Group 3 medulloblastoma accounts for 25% of diagnoses and typically arises in infants and young children. Group 3 tumors occur twice as frequently in males. This subgroup was associated with high rates of metastasis at the initial presentation.

Classic morphology is the most common histopathologic subtype; however, LC/A histology occurs in Group 3 more than the other molecular subgroups. This subgroup has the worst prognosis of all the molecular subgroups, with certain molecular features such as MYC amplification associated with dismal outcomes. Compared to WNT and SHH tumors, the molecular underpinnings of the remaining subgroups are less clearly defined. Group 3 tumors are highly aneuploid. Among this subgroup's most frequent cytogenetic events are the presence of isochromosome 17 q (i17q), chromosomes 1q and 7 gains, and chromosomes 8,10q, and 16 q losses.

Group 4 Medulloblastoma is the most common subgroup, accounting for 35–40% of all medulloblastoma diagnoses. This subgroup has the strongest male predilection, occurring over three times more commonly in males. Group 4 tumors are present across all age ranges, although they are relatively rare in infants. Peak incidence occurs in middle to late childhood. Most of Group 4 tumors have classic histology; however, a handful demonstrate DN or LC/A histology. Metastasis is present at diagnosis in approximately one-third of cases. This subgroup is considered to have an intermediate prognosis. Group 4 tumors appear to have transcriptional programs resembling unipolar brush cells and glutamatergic cerebellar nuclei, suggesting that progenitor cells within these lineages are the cells of origin for this subgroup. SHH Medulloblastoma accounts for approximately 30% of medulloblastoma diagnoses; however, it is the most common subtype among infant and adult patients but is less common during childhood and adolescence. The sex distribution is approximately even, with a slight male predominance. The histopathologic appearance of SHH tumors is variable, with all subtypes reported in this subgroup. Clinical characteristics, including histopathologic features, rate of metastasis, and prognosis, are variable based on patient age and molecular features, such as TP53 mutation status. Genetic predisposition syndromes have provided important insights into the role of the SHH signaling pathway in this subgroup, and genetic counseling remains an important diagnostic consideration in these patients, with up to 40% of pediatric cases occurring in patients with a cancer predisposition syndrome. Patients with Gorlin syndrome, an autosomal dominant condition that predisposes to the development of basal cell carcinoma, medulloblastoma, and other cancerous and noncancerous tumors, harbor germline mutations in SHH pathway genes, including PTCH1 and SUFU. Both of these genes are inhibitors of downstream SHH pathway activation. Mutation in these genes results in constitutive, ligand-independent activation of the SHH pathway, which normally regulates granule cell precursor proliferation in the developing cerebellum.

Author details

Parisa Zafari[1*] and Amir Azarhomayoun[2]

1 Faculty of Medicine, Department of Neurosurgery, Shahid Beheshti University of Medical Sciences, Tehran, Iran

2 Faculty of Medicine, Department of Neurosurgery, Tehran University of Medical Sciences, Tehran, Iran

*Address all correspondence to: parisazafari@yahoo.com

References

[1] Mahapatra S, Amsbaugh MJ. Medulloblastoma. In: StatPearls [Internet]. Treasure Island (FL): StatPearls Publishing; Jan 2024. Available from: https://www.ncbi.nlm.nih.gov/books/NBK431069/ [Updated 2023 Jun 26]

[2] Kijima N, Kanemura Y. Molecular Classification of Medulloblastoma. Neurologia Medico-Chirurgica (Tokyo). 15 Nov 2016;**56**(11):687-697. DOI: 10.2176/nmc.ra.2016-0016. Epub 2016 May 26. PMID: 27238212; PMCID: PMC5221779

[3] Vinchon M, Leblond P. Medulloblastoma: Clinical presentation. Neurochirurgie. Feb 2021;**67**(1):23-27. DOI: 10.1016/j.neuchi.2019.04.006. Epub 2019 Sep 5. PMID: 31494131

[4] Jallo GI. Medulloblastoma: Clinical presentation: History, physical, causes. In: Nelson SL, editor. 2022. Available from: https://emedicine.medscape.com/article/1181219-overview [Updated: Sep 27, 2022]

[5] Northcott PA, Dubuc A, Pfister S, Taylor MD. Molecular subgroups of MB. Expert Review of Neurotherapeutics. 2012;**12**(7):871-884

[6] Yeom KW, Mobley BC, Lober RM, Andre JB, Partap S, Vogel H, et al. Distinctive MRI features of pediatric medulloblastoma subtypes. American Journal of Roentgenology. 2013;**200**(4):895-903

[7] Fruehwald-Pallamar J, Puchner SB, R ossi A, Garre ML, Cama A, Koelblinger C, et al. Magnetic resonance imaging spectrum of medulloblastoma. Neuroradiology. 2011;**53**:387-396

[8] Perreault S, Ramaswamy V, Achrol AS, Chao K, Liu TT, Shih D, et al. MRI surrogates for molecular subgroups of medulloblastoma. American Journal of Neuroradiology. 2014;**35**(7):1263-1269

[9] Meyers SP, Wildenhain SL, Chang JK, Bourekas EC, Beattie PF, Korones DN, et al. Postoperative evaluation for disseminated medulloblastoma involving the spine: Contrast-enhanced MR findings, CSF cytologic analysis, timing of disease occurrence, and patient outcomes. American Journal of Neuroradiology. 2000;**21**(9):1757-1765

[10] Fouladi M, Gajjar A, Boyett JM, Walter AW, Thompson SJ, Merchant TE, et al. Comparison of CSF cytology and spinal magnetic resonance imaging in the detection of leptomeningeal disease in pediatric medulloblastoma or primitive neuroectodermal tumor. Journal of Clinical Oncology. 1999;**17**(10):3234-3237

[11] Gajjar A, Hernan R, Kocak M, Fuller C, Lee Y, McKinnon PJ, et al. Clinical, histopathologic, and molecular markers of prognosis: Toward a new disease risk stratification system for medulloblastoma. Journal of Clinical Oncology. 2004;**22**(6):984-993

[12] Ko Y, Gwak HS, Park EY, Joo J, Lee YJ, Lee SH, et al. Association of MRI findings with clinical characteristics and prognosis in patients with leptomeningeal carcinomatosis from non-small cell lung cancer. Journal of Neuro-Oncology. 2019;**143**:553-562

[13] Mirian C, Thastrup M, Mathiasen R, Schmiegelow K, Olsen JV, Østergaard O. Mass spectrometry-based proteomics of cerebrospinal fluid in pediatric central nervous system malignancies: A systematic review with meta-analysis of individual patient data. Fluids and Barriers of the CNS. 2024;**21**(1):1-17

[14] Ellison DW, Dalton J, Kocak M, Nicholson SL. MB: Clinicopathological correlates of SHH, WNT, and non-SHH/WNT molecular subgroups. Acta Neuropathologica. 2011;**121**(3):381-396

[15] Louis DN, Perry A, Reifenberger G, von Deimling A, Figarella-Branger D, Cavenee WK, et al. The 2016 World Health Organization classification of tumors of the central nervous system: A summary. Acta Neuropathologica. Jun 2016;**131**(6):803-820. DOI: 10.1007/s00401-016-1545-1. Epub 2016 May 9. PMID: 27157931

[16] Ostrom QT, Price M, Neff C, Cioffi G, Waite KA, Kruchko C, et al. CBTRUS statistical report: Primary brain and other central nervous system tumors diagnosed in the United States in 2016—2020. Neuro-Oncology. 2023;**25**(Suppl. 4):iv1-iv99

[17] Millard NE, De Braganca KC. Medulloblastoma. Journal of Child Neurology. 2016;**31**(12):1341-1353

[18] Massimino M, Biassoni V, Gandola L, Garrè ML, Gatta G, Giangaspero F, et al. Childhood medulloblastoma. Critical Reviews in Oncology/Hematology. 2016;**105**:35-51

[19] Liu Y, Xiao B, Li S, Liu J. Risk factors for survival in patients with medulloblastoma: A systematic review and meta-analysis. Frontiers in Oncology. 2022;**12**:827054

[20] Hovestadt V, Jones DTW, Picelli S, et al. Decoding the regulatory landscape of MB using DNA methylation profiling. Nature Communications. 2014;**5**:5069

[21] Bloch O, Cha S, Lapuk AV, et al. Targeting the immune microenvironment in MB: Novel immunotherapeutic approaches and implications for prognosis. Neuro-Oncology. 2020;**22**(1):3-15

[22] Klein-Gitelman MS, Kredich DW, Smith L, et al. Treatment-related toxicities in MB patients and their impact on long-term prognosis. Journal of Pediatric Oncology Nursing. 2012;**29**(1):42-52

[23] Lam S, Reddy GD, Lin Y, Jea A. Management of hydrocephalus in children with posterior fossa tumors. Surgical Neurology International. 23 Jul 2015;**6**(Suppl 11):S346-S348. DOI: 10.4103/2152-7806.161413. PMID: 26236555; PMCID: PMC4521311

[24] William J, Charles H. Schmidek and Sweet, Operative Neurosurgical Techniques. 7th ed. Jacksonville, Florida; 2022. pp. 19103-12899

[25] Ebrahim KS, Toubar AF. Telovelar approach versus transvermian approach in management of fourth ventricular tumors. Egyptian Journal of Neurosurgery. 2019;**34**:10. DOI: 10.1186/s41984-019-0036-9

[26] Ntenti C, Lallas K, Papazisis G. Clinical histological, and molecular prognostic factors in childhood medulloblastoma. 2023;**13**:1915. DOI: 10.3390/diagnostic 13111915

[27] Luther EM, Petridis AK, Dietz K, et al. Surgical site infections after posterior fossa brain surgery: A retrospective single-center analysis of incidence and risk factors. Acta Neurochirurgica. 2015;**157**(9):1631-1635

[28] Kumar R, Delaney H, Liverman CT, et al. Cerebrospinal fluid leaks after posterior fossa surgery in pediatric patients: Incidence, risk factors, and management outcomes. Child's Nervous System. 2018;**34**(7):1233-1240

[29] McCutcheon IE, Prabhu VC, McMahon JT, et al. Management of postoperative hydrocephalus following posterior fossa tumor resections in pediatric patients. Journal of Neurosurgery: Pediatrics. 2017;**19**(1):84-91

[30] Aydin K, Tang S, Weng J, et al. Cerebellar mutism syndrome in children post posterior fossa surgery: A comprehensive review of the literature. Child's Nervous System. 2019;**35**(9):1495-1502

[31] Tucha O, Smely C, Preier M, et al. Preoperative and postoperative cognitive functioning in patients with MB. Child's Nervous System. 2015;**31**(12):2079-2084

[32] Winn HR. Youmans and Winn Neurological Surgery E-Book: 4 – Volume. 8th ed. Netherlands: Elsevier Health Sciences; 2022

[33] Maier H, Dalianis T, Kostopoulou ON. New approaches in targeted therapy for medulloblastoma in children. Anticancer Research. 2021;**41**:1715-1726. DOI: 10.21873/anticancers.14936

Chapter 3

Pathology of Medulloblastoma: Morphologic Features and Molecular Classification

Thomas W. Smith

Abstract

This chapter presents an overview of the pathology of medulloblastoma. Historical aspects relating to the origin of medulloblastoma are briefly summarized. The current definition of medulloblastoma presented in the 2021 World Health Organization (WHO) Classification of Tumors of the Central Nervous System is discussed. This is followed by a description of the major gross and microscopic (histologic) features of medulloblastoma, and histologic criteria for the four major WHO subtypes. The role of immunohistochemistry in the classification of medulloblastoma is reviewed. The third part of the chapter focuses on the molecular classification of medulloblastoma as currently delineated in the 2021 WHO classification of Central Nervous System (CNS) tumors. This section presents in detail the methodology and criteria forming the basis of the molecular classification and how the different molecular groups correlate with the histologic subtypes and their immunohistochemical features. When appropriate, the clinical features relating to each molecular group are briefly discussed.

Keywords: medulloblastoma, histopathology, immunohistochemistry, molecular groups, methylation profiling

1. Introduction

Medulloblastoma is defined as a densely cellular "small blue cell tumor" that exclusively arises in the posterior fossa, primarily the cerebellum. In the 2021 World Health Organization (WHO) Classification of Tumors of the Central Nervous System (CNS), medulloblastoma is included within the general category of *CNS embryonal tumors* [1]. Although medulloblastomas may share some histological features with other CNS embryonal tumors, they are considered a unique tumor entity by virtue of their anatomic site of origin, histopathology, and molecular features.

Medulloblastoma has been traditionally classified as a CNS WHO grade 4 tumor, which still applies in the 2021 WHO classification [1]. This tumor grade is appropriate since it most accurately reflects the true biological behavior of the tumor. However, effective treatments that are now available have resulted in more favorable clinical outcomes and survival times, especially in cases aligned with specific molecular subgroups.

2. Historical background

2.1 Origin of medulloblastoma

The origin of the term "medulloblastoma" and how its usage has evolved over time is important in understanding the histopathology and current classification of the tumor. Medulloblastoma was first characterized by Cushing and Bailey in 1924 as a rapidly growing cerebellar tumor with a relatively poor prognosis [2, 3]. It was initially classified as a type of glioma and designated "spongioblastoma cerebelli" but was later changed to "medulloblastoma" to avoid confusion with other gliomas having a similar descriptive name [4]. Their classification of gliomas assumed that these tumors developed from undifferentiated neuroepithelial cells located in the medullary plate that could differentiate into spongioblasts, medulloblasts, and/or neuroblasts [3, 4]. This schema was based on a comparison of the histology of the various glioma types to their histologically normal counterparts in fetal and adult brains using metallic impregnation methods. Thus, the tumor designated as medulloblastoma was considered to be composed of primitive cells resembling rests of undifferentiated embryonal cells that were located in the roof of the fourth ventricle – these cells were referred to as "medulloblasts" [3]. The histologic uniqueness of this putative cell type further defined medulloblastoma as having an exclusive origin in the cerebellum.

2.2 Primitive neuroectodermal tumor (PNET)

In subsequent years, medulloblastoma became well-established as a uniquely cerebellar tumor with a characteristic histologic appearance. However, in 1973, Hart and Earle [5] first applied the term "primitive neuroectodermal tumor" to a series of CNS tumors (including medulloblastoma) having similar histologic features, and in the early 1980s, Rorke [6] expanded this concept and proposed an alternative classification based on the premise that all CNS tumors composed of undifferentiated neuroepithelial cells (as determined by the histologic and immunohistochemical methods then available) could be grouped together irrespective of their anatomic location. A basic assumption of this classification was that the neoplastic transformation of primitive neuroepithelial cells in the subependymal zones in all CNS regions would result in the same general tumor type. "Primitive neuroectodermal tumor" or PNET was thus established as the preferred term for this category of tumors. Medulloblastoma for example would now be classified as "cerebellar PNET". However, as more refined immunohistochemical and molecular data became available, it became clear that CNS tumors designated as "PNET" had a wide range of cellular origins and biological behaviors. In the most recent WHO classification of CNS tumors, the term "PNET" has been replaced by the more generic term "CNS embryonal tumor", which encompasses several specific entities as defined by modern histologic and molecular techniques [7]. Importantly medulloblastoma has been retained as the primary diagnostic category for histologically and molecular-defined tumors that arise in the cerebellum [1]. Removal of the CNS PNET category from the WHO classification also resolved confusion with peripheral (non-CNS) PNETs, which have different cellular origins, molecular biology, and clinical behavior.

2.3 WHO classification of CNS tumors

The most recent WHO classifications have retained *medulloblastoma* as the designated term for CNS embryonal tumors arising in the posterior fossa/cerebellum that have the characteristic morphologic and molecular features of this tumor. In the 2021 WHO classification, medulloblastoma is grouped into two categories: histologically-defined medulloblastoma and molecularly-defined medulloblastoma [1]. Ideally, the pathologic diagnosis of medulloblastoma should incorporate both histologic and molecular features within a unitary "integrated diagnosis", as WHO recommends for many other CNS tumors [7]. The advantage of this approach is that it better addresses the biological and clinical behavior of medulloblastoma and helps guide approaches to therapy. However, molecular studies often take an extended time to complete, and in the case of medulloblastoma, they may also require referral to an outside testing laboratory. Thus, in many institutions, a histological diagnosis of medulloblastoma is initially rendered with the integrated or molecular diagnosis as an addendum to the pathology report.

3. Morphologic features of medulloblastoma

3.1 Gross pathology

Descriptions of the gross pathology of medulloblastoma have been largely derived from postmortem examinations or observations made at the time of surgical resection. The gross appearance of medulloblastoma generally correlates well with the radiological features of the tumor; however, there are no gross features that are entirely specific to this tumor. At the time of surgery, the tumor is typically described as having a soft, fleshy, gray-pink appearance and may occasionally have small cysts, areas of hemorrhage and/or necrosis in some regions [8]. Calcifications are not present. The tumor may grossly appear to be relatively well-circumscribed (a feature also noted on radiologic imaging); however, microscopically the tumor will almost always show some infiltration into the adjacent parenchyma [9]. Tumors located in the lateral cerebellar hemisphere may have desmoplastic/nodular cytoarchitecture (described below) in association with increased amounts of connective tissue, which may impart a firm character to the tumor. Although medulloblastoma is defined as a tumor originating within the cerebellum, it can extend into the fourth ventricle and may present as an intraventricular mass. Rostral extension into the pineal region may also occur; however, in most cases, radiographic studies and/or surgical observation will allow differentiation from a primary pineal neoplasm. Since medulloblastomas (in common with other CNS embryonal tumors) are capable of intraventricular and leptomeningeal spread, they can present as lesions in other regions of the CNS, in particular the spinal cord.

3.2 Histopathology

3.2.1 Light microscopic features and histologic subtypes

The WHO classification recognizes four histological subtypes: classic medulloblastoma, desmoplastic/nodular medulloblastoma, medulloblastoma with extensive nodularity, and large cell/anaplastic medulloblastoma [8, 10]. An attempt has been made to match these histologic subtypes to the molecular groups described below; however, it should be emphasized that the morphologic features of these subtypes are not sufficient to identify or confirm a specific molecular group or subgroup.

3.2.2 Classic medulloblastoma

This is the most common histologic pattern of medulloblastoma and is characterized as a densely cellular undifferentiated "small blue cell" tumor [8, 10]. The tumor cells are small and consist almost entirely of irregular, densely hyperchromatic nuclei (dark blue on H&E stains) with very little, if any, visible cytoplasm (**Figure 1A**). Homer Wright (neuroblastic) rosettes (**Figure 1B**) may be present, but unlike peripheral neuroblastoma, they are relatively infrequent and found in less than 40% of cases. Some tumor cells may appear to have delicate fibrillary processes. Some classic medulloblastomas may have less densely cellular nodular zones, but unlike the desmoplastic/nodular subtype, the nodules lack desmoplasia (reticulin deposition at the periphery of nodules). However, if a classic medulloblastoma invades leptomeninges, desmoplasia may be present but in a non-perinodular configuration. Mitoses are present but are sometimes difficult to visualize, and apoptotic tumor cells are often apparent. Tumor vascularity may be high; however, microvascular proliferation (a common feature of high-grade glioma) is not a typical feature of medulloblastoma. Some tumors may have confluent or geographic areas of necrosis; however, the necrotic foci are usually non-palisading.

3.2.3 Desmoplastic/nodular medulloblastoma

This histologic subtype is characterized by its nodular architecture and perinodular desmoplasia (**Figure 2**) [8, 10]. Since both features are required for the diagnosis,

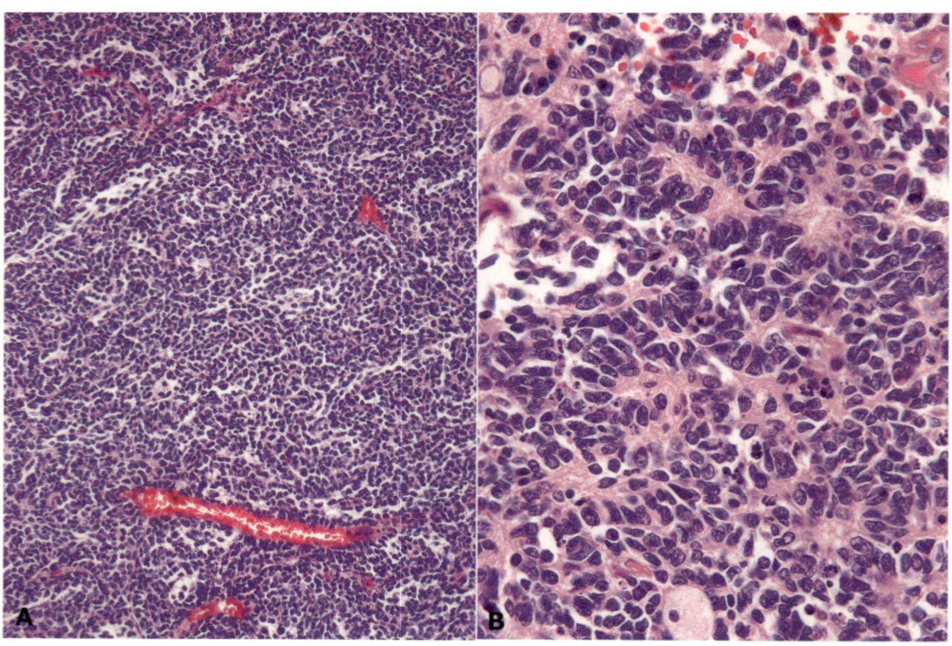

Figure 1.
Classic medulloblastoma. (A) The tumor is densely cellular and consists of small cells with irregular hyperchromatic nuclei and little or no visible cytoplasm. Nodular architecture is not present. H&E x10. (B) Homer Wright (neuroblastic) rosettes may be present in some classic medulloblastomas. H&E x40.

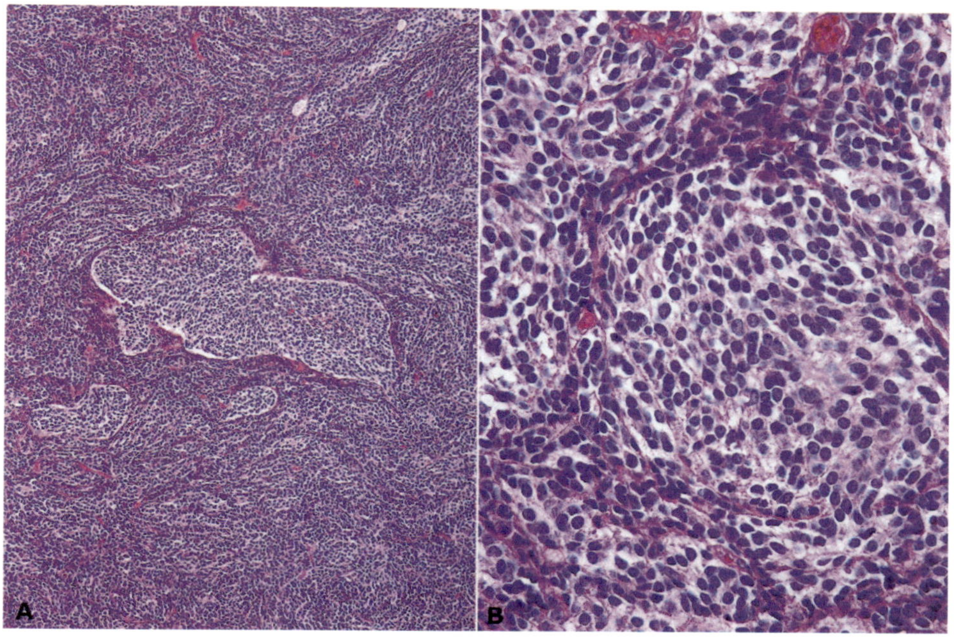

Figure 2.
Desmoplastic/nodular medulloblastoma. (A) Most regions of the tumor have an easily discernable nodular appearance, which is highlighted by the presence of peri-nodular deposition of reticulin and collagen. Homer Wright rosettes are not present in this subtype. H&E x10. (B) The nodules are less densely cellular compared to classic medulloblastoma. H&E x40.

it is imperative to perform a reticulin stain to identify them. The nodules can vary in size but are readily identified by their less dense cellularity and perinodular deposition of reticulin and collagen. The peripheral zones of the nodules are more densely cellular and consist of less-differentiated cells with pleomorphic hyperchromatic nuclei and apoptotic cells. These zones will show increased mitotic activity and an elevated Ki-67 labeling index. Homer Wright's rosettes are not present. The desmoplastic/nodular histologic subtype shows a high correlation with the SHH-activated and TP53-wildtype molecular group [11].

3.2.4 Medulloblastoma with extensive nodularity

This tumor has histologic features that resemble the desmoplastic/nodular subtype but differ from the latter by their less conspicuous perinodular reticulin/collagen deposition and expanded lobular architecture (**Figure 3**) [8, 10]. Coalescence of nodules may result in a streaming pattern. The relatively hypocellular nodules have a population of small round cells with fibrillary cytoplasm that show neurocytic differentiation by immunohistochemistry. The interlobular regions show increased cellularity, mitotic activity, and elevated Ki-67 labeling indices.

3.2.5 Large cell/anaplastic medulloblastoma

This histologic subtype is characterized by the presence of large cell and/or anaplastic morphology (**Figure 4**) [8, 10]. In previous WHO classifications, these tumors

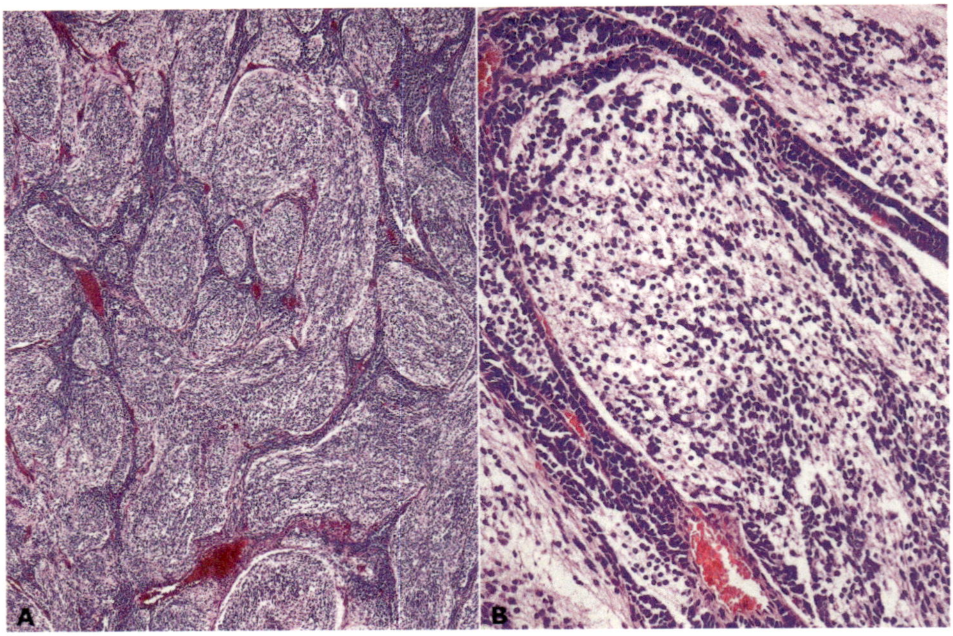

Figure 3.
Medulloblastoma with extensive nodularity. (A) The histologic appearance of this tumor closely resembles the desmoplastic/nodular subtype but shows more prominent nodular architecture. Some coalescent nodules have a streaming appearance. H&E x4. (B) The interior of the nodules is relatively hypocellular and shows neurocytic differentiation by immunohistochemistry. The interlobular regions show higher cellularity, mitotic activity, and increased Ki-67 labeling. Homer Wright rosettes are not present. H&E x20.

were grouped into two separate phenotypic categories but are now combined within a single group, since their histologic features often overlap. The large cell pattern is characterized by tumor cells that are larger than usually seen in the other histologic subtypes and have large, variably pleomorphic nuclei and prominent nucleoli. In the anaplastic pattern, the tumor cells show increased mitotic activity, many apoptotic cells, and other histologic features such as nuclear molding, cytoplasmic pseudoinclusions, and tumor cell wrapping. In comparison to the other medulloblastoma subtypes, the large cell/anaplastic variant appears to be associated with more aggressive clinical behavior [8, 10]. Classic medulloblastomas that have focal areas of increased anaplasia should not be reclassified as large cell/anaplastic tumors if this is not the predominant histologic pattern. However, the presence of anaplastic foci in the tumor should be mentioned to alert clinicians of the possibility of more aggressive behavior.

3.2.6 Medulloblastomas with non-WHO designated histologic patterns

Several rare but distinctive morphologic patterns of divergent differentiation may occur in medulloblastoma: medulloblastoma with myogenic differentiation ("medullomyoblastoma") and medulloblastoma with melanocytic differentiation ("melanocytic medulloblastoma") [10]. Either pattern may arise in any of the WHO-recognized histologic subtypes. Immunohistochemistry may be needed to identify myogenic or melanocytic cells when they are not readily identified by routine histology [10]. There is currently no evidence that the presence of divergent differentiation alters the major histologic or molecular classification of medulloblastoma.

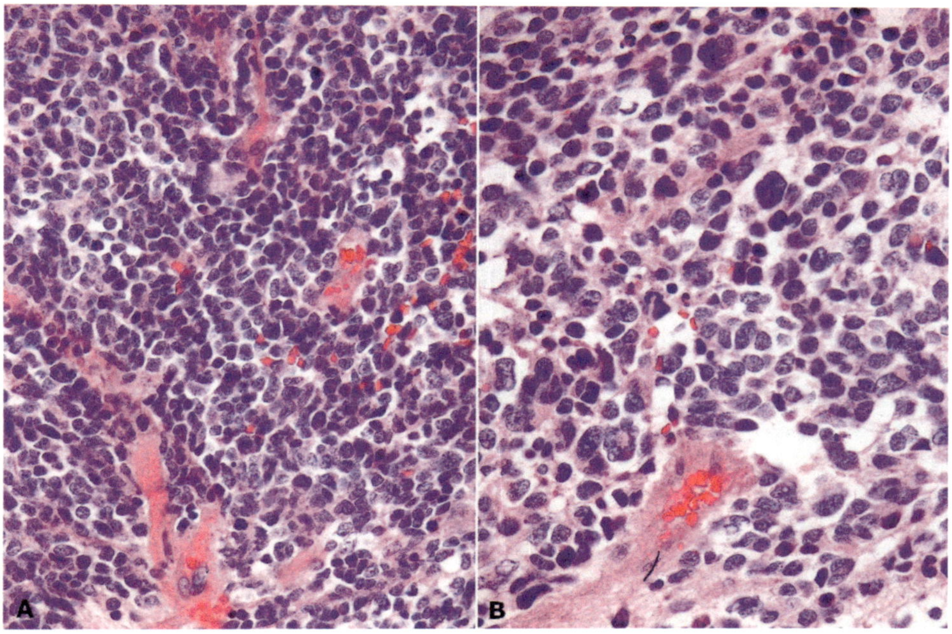

Figure 4.
Large cell/anaplastic medulloblastoma. (A) The tumor cells are larger than usually seen in the other histologic subtypes and exhibit greater cytologic atypia. Nodular architecture and Homer Wright rosettes are not present. H&E x20. (B) Higher magnification highlights the increased cell size, marked nuclear pleomorphism, apoptotic bodies, and mitoses. H&E x60.

3.3 Immunohistochemistry (IHC): diagnostic considerations

There are no immunohistochemical markers that are entirely specific for medulloblastoma; however, an IHC panel directed toward antigens that are frequently present or absent in this tumor can be used to confirm the diagnosis and to exclude tumors that may histologically mimic medulloblastoma [8, 10]. Most medulloblastomas will show reactivity for the neuronal markers synaptophysin and/or NeuN but are less often positive for neurofilament proteins. Tumor cells may rarely express GFAP ("spongioblastic differentiation"); however, it is more common to find reactive GFAP-positive astrocytes in the tumor. This feature should not be interpreted as evidence of glial differentiation. IHC markers commonly used in the diagnosis of glial tumors (e.g., IDH1, OLIG2, and EMA) should be negative. Since atypical teratoid rhabdoid tumors often share histologic features with medulloblastoma, IHC for SMARCB1/INI1 should always be performed [12]. Other CNS embryonal tumors with overlapping histologic features may require additional tumor-specific IHC (e.g., embryonal tumor with multilayered rosettes – LIN28A [13] and pineoblastoma – CRX [14]). Embryonal cerebellar tumors that cannot be reliably classified by IHC will require molecular testing including DNA methylation profiling [15]. Surrogate IHC markers (discussed below) have been used to classify medulloblastoma into molecular groups [10], but this approach has some limitations and has been largely replaced by methylation profiling as the preferred method for molecular classification. IHC may be needed to exclude poorly differentiated or small cell carcinoma or lymphoma, especially in older patients with cerebellar tumors that may histologically resemble medulloblastoma.

4. Molecular classification of medulloblastoma

Medulloblastomas are classified into four major molecular groups: Wingless/INT1 (WNT)-activated, sonic hedgehog (SHH)-activated (includes TP53-wildtype and TP53-mutant groups), non-WNT/non-SHH group 3, and non-WNT/non-SHH group 4 [1]. The two non-WNT/non-SHH groups are usually combined into a single group. The SHH-activated group can further be divided into four subgroups, and the non-WNT/non-SHH group can be divided into eight subgroups by DNA methylation or transcriptome profiling [1]. The molecular classification of medulloblastoma was initially developed using transcription profiling, which was based on shared RNA expression patterns detected by transcription array and RNA sequencing. More recently, the wider availability of DNA methylation profiling has made this the preferred method for the molecular classification of medulloblastoma. Molecular classification based on immunohistochemistry and/or DNA sequencing has also been used but is limited in its ability to reliably detect all tumor groups [10].

4.1 Medulloblastoma, WNT-activated

WNT-activated tumors account for approximately 10–15% of all medulloblastomas [10, 16]. They most often occur in children between ages 7 and 14, with a slight predominance in females, but about 15–20% occur in adults. Tumors in this molecular group usually arise near the midline and can often involve the cerebellar peduncle or brainstem. Molecular studies suggest that WNT-activated tumors originate from progenitor cells in the lower rhombic lip in the dorsal brainstem [17]. The majority of WNT-activated medulloblastomas belong histologically to the *classic subtype*. The prognosis of WNT-activated medulloblastomas occurring in children has generally been quite favorable [10, 16].

4.1.1 Diagnostic considerations

Activation of the WNT pathway can be demonstrated by IHC for β catenin, which shows diffuse or patchy nuclear reactivity [16]. Other medulloblastoma subtypes may show cytoplasmic but not nuclear immunoreactivity for β catenin. Molecular testing will show CTNNB1 exon three mutations and loss or partial loss of chromosome six in about 85–90% of cases [16]. Tumors lacking this molecular profile may show germline APC mutations [16]. As mentioned above, methylation profiling remains the preferred method for identifying medulloblastoma molecular groups and subgroups.

4.2 Medulloblastoma, SHH-activated

SHH-activated tumors account for approximately 30% of medulloblastomas [10, 11]. They have a bimodal age and location presentation: those occurring in infants most often arise in the cerebellar vermis, whereas those in older children and adults arise mainly in the cerebellar hemispheres [11]. SHH-activated medulloblastomas are thought to arise from progenitor cells located in the cerebellar external granule cell layer [18]. Several hereditary tumor syndromes are associated with this molecular group (see below). The 2021 WHO classification further divides SHH-activated medulloblastomas into two major molecular categories: SHH-activated and TP53-wildtype, and SHH-activated and TP53-mutant [11, 19]. They differ primarily in their predominant histologic subtype, associated tumor syndromes, and clinical behavior.

4.2.1 SHH-activated and TP53-wildtype medulloblastoma

The predominant histologic subtypes in this group are desmoplastic/nodular medulloblastoma and medulloblastoma with extensive nodularity [11]. The hereditary tumor syndrome most often associated with this subgroup is the nevoid basal cell carcinoma syndrome (Gorlin syndrome), most often due to inactivating germline mutations in PTCH1 [11]. Medulloblastomas occurring in infants with a nodular/desmoplastic or extensively nodular cytoarchitecture are SSH-activated and TP53-wildtype (mainly SHH subgroups 1 and 2) and have a generally favorable prognosis [11].

4.2.2 SHH-activated and TP53-mutant medulloblastoma

The predominant histologic subtype in this molecular group is large cell/anaplastic, which aligns with the SHH-3 subgroup [19]. Approximately half are associated with germline mutations in TP53 (Li-Fraumeni syndrome) [19]. Children (non-infant) and adults with SHH-activated, TP53 mutant, and MYCN-amplified tumors generally have a poor prognosis [20].

4.2.3 Diagnostic considerations

Although methylation profiling is the preferred method for classification of all molecular groups, IHC can sometimes be used to differentiate the SHH-activated group from other medulloblastoma molecular groups and to identify the presence of a TP53 mutation [10, 11, 16, 19]. SHH-activated tumors express both GAB1 and YAP1 but do not show nuclear staining for β catenin, whereas WNT-activated tumors express YAP1 but not GAB1 and show nuclear expression for β catenin. Non-WNT/non-SHH tumors do not express GAB1, YAP1, or nuclear reactivity for β catenin. Widespread and strong nuclear immunoreactivity for p53 almost always reflects the presence of a TP53 mutation; however, cases showing low/equivocal or absent p53 immunoreactivity will require molecular profiling. Molecular sequencing is also needed to demonstrate MYCN amplification or specific SHH pathway mutations (e.g., PTCH1, SMO, and SUFU) that may yield additional prognostic information [10].

4.3 Medulloblastoma, non-WNT/non-SHH

This molecular group is a heterogeneous and complex category of medulloblastoma that was initially subdivided into two major molecular groups – groups 3 and 4 [1, 21]. DNA methylation profiling has more recently divided the group 3/4 tumors into eight distinct molecular subgroups [1]. These tumors usually arise in the midline of the cerebellum, often filling the fourth ventricle [10]. A significant proportion of patients in this molecular group present with distant CNS metastases at the time of diagnosis [10, 21]. Group 3 tumors occur most often in infants and young children, and group 4 in older children and adults [10]. Groups 3 and 4 tumors comprise approximately 25% and 40%, respectively, of all medulloblastomas and tend to have the worst prognosis of all molecular subgroups [10, 21]. This molecular group is not associated with known hereditary tumor syndromes. MYC amplification is most often present in group 3 tumors and is associated with a poor outcome [21]. Non-WNT/non-SHH medulloblastomas are most often associated with the classic histologic subtype; however, the large cell/anaplastic subtype may also occur in both groups 3 and 4 and has a particular association with subgroup 2 [21].

4.3.1 Diagnostic considerations

Although immunohistochemistry can sometimes be used to differentiate WNT-activated and SHH-activated medulloblastomas from the non-WNT/non-SHH molecular group, the molecular classification of the eight group 3/4 subgroups requires methylation profiling, often combined with transcriptomic analysis [1]. These subgroups differ in their biological and molecular characteristics, clinical course, and prognostic significance [22].

5. Conclusion

The classification of medulloblastoma is based on both histopathologic and molecular features and is required for proper assessment of the biologic and clinical behavior of a given tumor, including prognosis and response to therapy. The features of the principle histopathologic subgroups and the current molecular classification have been reviewed. The histopathologic classification of medulloblastoma and importantly, their distinction from other CNS embryonal neoplasms can often be facilitated by immunohistochemistry. DNA methylation profiling is now the preferred method to correctly classify histologically challenging CNS embryonal tumors and to establish the molecular classification of medulloblastoma.

Conflict of interest

The author declares no conflict of interest.

Author details

Thomas W. Smith
Department of Pathology, University of Massachusetts Medical School, Worcester, Massachusetts, USA

*Address all correspondence to: thomas.smith@umassmemorial.org

References

[1] Ellison DW, Taylor MD. Medulloblastoma: introduction. In: WHO Classification of Tumours Editorial Board, editor. WHO Classification of Tumours. Central Nervous System Tumours. 5th ed. Lyon: IARC Press; 2021. pp. 200-202

[2] Kunschner LJ. Harvey Cushing and Medulloblastoma. Archives of Neurology. 2002;**59**(4):642-645. DOI: 10.1001/archneur.59.4.642

[3] Juraschka K, Taylor MD. Medulloblastoma in the age of molecular subgroups: A review. Journal of Neurosurgery. Pediatrics. 2019;**24**(4): 353-363. DOI: 10.3171/2019.5.PEDS18381

[4] Ferguson S, Lesniak MS. Percival bailey and the classification of brain tumors. Neurosurgical Focus. 2005;**18**(4):e7. DOI: 10.3171/foc.2005.18.4.8

[5] Hart MN, Earle KM. Primitive neuroectodermal tumors of the brain in children. Cancer. 1973;**32**(4):890-897. DOI: 10.1002/1097-0142(197310)32:4 <890::aid-cncr2820320421>3.0.co;2-o

[6] Rorke LB. The cerebellar medulloblastoma and its relationship to primitive neuroectodermal tumors. Journal of Neuropathology and Experimental Neurology. 1983 Jan;**42**(1):1-15

[7] Louis DN, Perry A, Wesseling P, Brat DJ, Cree IA, Figarella-Branger D, et al. The 2021 WHO classification of Tumors of the central nervous system: A summary. Neuro-Oncology. 2021;**23**(8):1231-1251. DOI: 10.1093/neuonc/noab106

[8] Korshunov A, Ellison DW, Giangaspero F, Orr BA, Pietsch T, Taylor MD. Medulloblastoma, histologically defined. In: WHO Classification of Tumours Editorial Board, editor. WHO Classification of Tumours. Central Nervous System Tumours. 5th ed. Lyon: IARC Press; 2021. pp. 213-219

[9] Perreault S, Ramaswamy V, Achrol AS, Chao K, Liu TT, Shih D, et al. MRI surrogates for molecular subgroups of medulloblastoma. AJNR American Journal of Neuroradiology. 2014;**35**(7):1263-1269. DOI: 10.3174/ajnr.A3990

[10] Orr BA. Pathology, diagnostics, and classification of medulloblastoma. Brain Pathology. 2020 May;**30**(3):664-678. DOI: 10.1111/bpa.12837

[11] Ellison DW, Clifford SC, Kaur K, Korshunov A, Northcott PA, Taylor MD. Medulloblastoma, SHH-activated and TP53-wildtype. In: WHO Classification of Tumours Editorial Board, editor. WHO Classification of Tumours. Central Nervous System Tumours. 5th ed. Lyon: IARC Press; 2021. pp. 205-207

[12] Haberler C, Hasselblatt M, Huang A, Judkins AR, Kool M, Wesseling P. Atypical teratoid/rhabdoid tumour. In: WHO Classification of Tumours Editorial Board, editor. WHO Classification of Tumours. Central Nervous System Tumours. 5th ed. Lyon: IARC Press; 2021. pp. 221-225

[13] Korshunov A, Fuller GN, Haberler C, Huang A, Kool M, Sturm D, et al. Embryonal tumour with multilayered rosettes. In: WHO Classification of Tumours Editorial Board, editor. WHO Classification of Tumours. Central Nervous System Tumours. 5th ed. Lyon: IARC Press; 2021. pp. 228-231

[14] Hasselblatt M, Huang A, Jones DTW, Orr BA, Snuderl M, Vasiljevic A. Pineoblastoma. In: WHO Classification of Tumours Editorial Board, editor. WHO Classification of Tumours. Central Nervous System Tumours. 5th ed. Lyon: IARC Press; 2021. pp. 249-252

[15] Wesseling P, Pfister SM. Other CNS embryonal tumours: Introduction. In: WHO Classification of Tumours Editorial Board, editor. WHO Classification of Tumours. Central Nervous System Tumours. 5th ed. Lyon: IARC Press; 2021. p. 220

[16] Ellison DW, Clifford SC, Kaur K, Korshunov A, Northcott PA, Taylor MD. Medulloblastoma, WNT-activated. In: WHO Classification of Tumours Editorial Board, editor. WHO Classification of Tumours. Central Nervous System Tumours. 5th ed. Lyon: IARC Press; 2021. pp. 203-204

[17] Gibson P, Tong Y, Robinson G, Thompson MC, Currle DS, Eden C, et al. Subtypes of medulloblastoma have distinct developmental origins. Nature. 2010;**468**(7327):1095-1099. DOI: 10.1038/nature09587

[18] Schüller U, Heine VM, Mao J, Kho AT, Dillon AK, Han YG, et al. Acquisition of granule neuron precursor identity is a critical determinant of progenitor cell competence to form Shh-induced medulloblastoma. Cancer Cell. 2008;**14**(2):123-134. DOI: 10.1016/j.ccr.2008.07.005

[19] Ellison DW, Clifford SC, Kaur K, Korshunov A, Northcott PA, Taylor MD. Medulloblastoma, SHH-activated and TP53-mutant. In: WHO Classification of Tumours Editorial Board, editor. WHO Classification of Tumours. Central Nervous System Tumours. 5th ed. Lyon: IARC Press; 2021. pp. 208-210

[20] Ramaswamy V, Nör C, Taylor MD. p53 and Meduloblastoma. Cold Springer Harbor Perspective Medicine. 2015;**6**(2):a026278. DOI: 10.1101/cshperspect.a026278, 10.1101/cshperspect.a029579

[21] Ellison DW, Clifford SC, Kaur K, Korshunov A, Northcott PA, Taylor MD. Medulloblastoma, non-WNT/non-SHH. In: WHO Classification of Tumours Editorial Board, editor. WHO Classification of Tumours. Central Nervous System Tumours. 5th ed. Lyon: IARC Press; 2021. pp. 211-212

[22] Korshunov A, Okonechnikov K, Schrimpf D, Tonn S, Mynarek M, Koster J, et al. Transcriptome analysis stratifies second-generation non-WNT/non-SHH medulloblastoma subgroups into clinically tractable subtypes. Acta Neuropathologica. 2023 Jun;**145**(6):829-842. DOI: 10.1007/s00401-023-02575-z

Chapter 4

Medulloblastoma: Systemic Chemotherapy and Future Applications of Chemoradiotherapy

Julia Hayden, Stefanie Lowas, Nura El-Haj, Naheed Usmani, Koren Smith, Matthew Iandoli, Fran Laurie, Maryann Bishop-Jodoin, Eric Ko and Paul Rava

Abstract

Medulloblastoma is the most common malignant brain tumor in children. Prognosis remains guarded in patients who at diagnosis are very young, have craniospinal metastatic disease, or after resection, have residual disease. Treatment incorporates chemotherapy and radiation therapy. Cancer survivors often have life-altering treatment effects. This chapter reviews clinical trials over the years and the efforts to improve survival and minimize sequelae along with challenges in performing clinical trials. Quality assurance of the radiation therapy provided worldwide monitors compliance. Advances in the risk stratification and targeted treatment based on the genomics and biology of medulloblastoma are highlighted in recent clinical trials. Through chemotherapy aligned with specific biomarkers, sophisticated radiation therapy strategies, and continued quality assurance, the future vision of managing medulloblastoma is presented.

Keywords: medulloblastoma, radiation therapy, chemotherapy, children, clinical trials, biomarker, precision therapy

1. Introduction

Although medulloblastoma (MB) will affect two patients for every million people per year, the disease remains the most common malignant brain tumor in children comprising 15% of primary brain tumors in children [1]. Forty percent (40%) of patients with MB are identified before the age of 5, with approximately 70% of patients identified before the age of 10. Prognosis remains guarded in patients who are exceptionally young at diagnosis (<36 months), patients with limited surgical resection with residual post-surgical disease, or patients with metastatic disease at presentation including disease in the cerebral spinal fluid axis. Because of the propensity of the disease to involve the cerebral fluid pathways, radiation therapy (RT) is delivered in this disease to the entire cranial spinal neuroaxis. There has been

IntechOpen

limited success when the RT volume and dose to target have been titrated; therefore, patients remain at risk for measurable sequelae of management despite treatment with curative intent, especially given the propensity of younger patients affected with this disease [2]. With cumulative survival rates at 20 years of 50% using traditional therapies including craniospinal radiation therapy (CSRT), efforts have been made in multiple clinical trial settings to improve tumor control and potentially address the development of sequelae by using more advanced technology RT coupled with systemic therapy. Because RT treats large segments of normal tissue including bone marrow reserves, integrating chemotherapy either before, during, or after RT has been challenging. Effort identifying a consistent and strategic pathway for the application and integration of systemic care in this patient population is the focus of several clinical trials. In this chapter, the chemotherapy management of patients with MB from a historical and protocol perspective is reviewed, as well as strategies for care for the next generation of clinical trials in this disease currently characterized by unique biomarker expression products. The future vision of modern systemic therapy aligned to specific biomarkers identified in subsets of patients affected with this disease will be presented.

2. Past and current management involving systemic therapy for medulloblastoma

From a historical perspective, surgery followed by postoperative RT to the neuroaxis including boost to the primary site of the disease including sites of metastatic disease in the central nervous system and spine had been considered a standard of care for patients with MB. It was recognized by early investigators that, despite clinical control of disease in selected patients, RT had the potential to impose significant neurocognitive, endocrine, hearing, and developmental sequelae as a consequence to curative management [3–6]. The sequelae can often be life altering for the cancer survivors and impose significant long-term changes in function for living with the consequence of management. The goal of introducing systemic therapy for these patients was to improve upon survival outcomes and potentially limit normal tissue sequelae imposed by higher-dose RT.

There have been challenges integrating chemotherapy with RT in these vulnerable patients. Although CSRT is highly effective, it imposes measurable acute and late effects due to the volume of normal tissue unintentionally included in the RT treatment field. Because disease has access to the cerebral spinal fluid pathways, the entire cranial and spinal neuroaxis is considered a clinical target volume and requires RT for microscopic and macroscopic disease control [7, 8]. In the initial RT strategy for treatment, the anatomy of the central nervous system and the neuroaxis became what we refer to today as the clinical target volume. Chemotherapy can have an additive effect to tumor control as well as impose acceleration of injury to tissues being irradiated. With the fluid pathways at risk for disease, the entire central nervous system, by default, receives treatment [7]. For patients, especially younger children affected by the disease, this can impose injury with consequence. For example, the temporal lobe and temporal bone mature at a later time point in development than other areas of the central nervous system; therefore, neurocognition, endocrine, auditory, processing, and verbal skills can be negatively impacted by therapy at a time point important for growth and development during adolescence [3–6]. Exit dose from thoracic spine fields can impose cardiopulmonary sequelae relative to field width size in an age-related manner with direct impact on growth and development of the spine as an additional problem. Exit dose can also influence bowel, renal, ovarian, and testicular function if dose is not managed as part of a conformal avoidance strategy. Vertebral body development and development of pelvis structures can likewise be influenced [9], especially in patients with high-risk features that require a higher dose to target, therefore leading to a higher dose to bone including joint spaces. Although the target volume for the RT boost plan can be titrated with confidence to spare normal tissue including the cochlea from high dose, studies to date have demonstrated that decreasing the dose to the cranial spinal axis, in selected favorable patients, cannot be safely accomplished for the general population. Therefore, even moving forward, protocols written for molecular-driven subsets of patients with this disease will require extended volume RT for the majority of patients, possibly excluding those with highly favorable features on biomarker analysis and the exceptionally young.

Chemotherapy application strategies have to be both comprehensive and thoughtful. Interdigitating chemotherapy either before, during, or after RT has to be accomplished in a manner that the patient receives the best of both disciplines and not the additive consequence of both therapies. Because of the complexity of interdigitating therapy as part of a composite treatment program with goals of improved tumor control and normal tissue outcome, studies have not uniformly shown benefits to combined modality therapy. Nevertheless, chemotherapy including the advent of biomarker-specific targeted therapy remains the best option to improve outcomes and balance the known effects of RT.

In an important historical paper written by Michiels and colleagues from the Netherlands in 2015, investigators identified seven retrospective and historical clinical trials for meta-analysis to determine the efficacy of treatment including and not including chemotherapy in patients treated for MB. The studies included 1080 patients and intended to review both event-free survival (EFS) and disease-free survival (DFS). As often the case with retrospective analysis, there were inconsistencies in applying metrics for disease progression, and essential information including stage at presentation and completion of surgical intervention was often less clear. Two of the studies without clear definition of disease progression revealed no statistical difference between those treated with chemotherapy and not treated with chemotherapy. In another study, improvements in the chemotherapy-treated patients were only evident during the course of treatment; however, the significance was no longer visible with longer follow-up. The review identified one retrospective clinical trial comparing standard-dose RT and reduced-dose RT coupled with chemotherapy without a difference in EFS or DFS between the groups. This trial did not evaluate quality of life nor had sub-group analysis. Multiple chemotherapy agents were used in these protocols and include cisplatin (CDDP), cyclophosphamide (CPM), vincristine (VCR), etoposide (VP-16), carboplatin, methotrexate (MTX), lomustine (CCNU), and topotecan. Chemotherapy was applied at multiple timepoints as part of the evolution of standard of care for this disease. Although the review has considerable strength and value, the review points to the need for trials to be conducted with rigor and discipline to optimize what we can learn from the trial and generate process improvements in clinical care for this vulnerable patient population. If outcomes for patients can be improved and applied directly into clinical care, the information from the trial must be trusted by the oncology clinical community. This is especially true in a disease such as MB, which requires hundreds of institutions to participate on a worldwide basis in order to accrue enough patients to trial and answer important study questions concerning both tumor control and normal tissue tolerance [10].

The National Clinical Trials Network (NCTN) of the National Cancer Institute (NCI) provides an extraordinary and robust administrative and quality assurance mechanism for the conduct of oncology-driven clinical trials. Data management centers coupled with important core services including the Imaging and Radiation Oncology Core (IROC) and tissue banks provide security that data will be acquired, processed, and maintained in a manner to support analysis of primary and secondary clinical trial endpoints in a rigorous and consistent manner. Data, including pathology objects, can be archived and repurposed for secondary analysis of additional study endpoints not anticipated at the time of the initial trial design. Through this prism and data management architecture, clinical trials are developed and vetted through NCI disease and discipline trial committees in order to (1) ask important and clinically relevant study questions and (2) support the infrastructure to ensure appropriate trial conduct and management. The Children's Oncology Group (COG) is one of the major clinical cooperative groups and is an outstanding resource for this purpose as it includes all of the necessary administrative and clinical tools necessary to manage hundreds of clinical trials and thousands of trial participants. During this next section, we will review how chemotherapy has been applied in protocol settings and what we can anticipate as a treatment strategy as we move toward molecular classification of the disease [11–13].

3. Chemotherapeutic strategy in medulloblastoma

Current approaches in the treatment of MB include both adjuvant and maintenance chemotherapy regimens and RT. Protocols are working to determine combination chemotherapy regimens that improve overall and progression-free survival (PFS), sensitize tumors to RT, and limit toxicities.

3.1 A9961

This study was an intergroup study involving the Children's Cancer Group (CCG) and the Pediatric Oncology Group (POG) prior to the merger of the groups into the COG. The study treated patients ages 3–21 with standard-risk MB who had negative cerebral spinal fluid and less than 1.5 cm^2 residual disease in the posterior fossa. Patients were treated to a dose of 23.4 Gy to the cranial spinal axis with a boost dose of 32.4 Gy to the anatomically defined posterior fossa generally with lateral fields and two-dimensional radiation planning techniques. The study tested if the use of post-RT application of cyclophosphamide would improve outcome compared to established regimens. This study enrolled 421 patients. After RT was completed, patients were randomized to treatment with either adjuvant CCNU (oral; 75 mg/m^2 on day 1), CDDP (75 mg/m^2 IV on day 1), and VCR (1.5 mg/m^2 IV bolus, max dose 2 mg on days 1, 7, 14) or adjuvant CPM (1000 IV mg/m^2 on days 21, 22), CDDP, and VCR (**Figure 1**). The overall survival at 5 years was 86%, and the overall 5-year EFS was 81%. The CCNU and CPM arm results were in similar PFS, overall survival, and toxicity. Ototoxicity was the most significant adverse event in both arms. Although likely a competing consequence from CDDP treatment, patients were treated with lateral-field RT for both primary management and the boost, therefore incorporating auditory structures including the cochlea in the treatment field receiving prescription dose, which affected hearing as a late effect in both study arms [15].

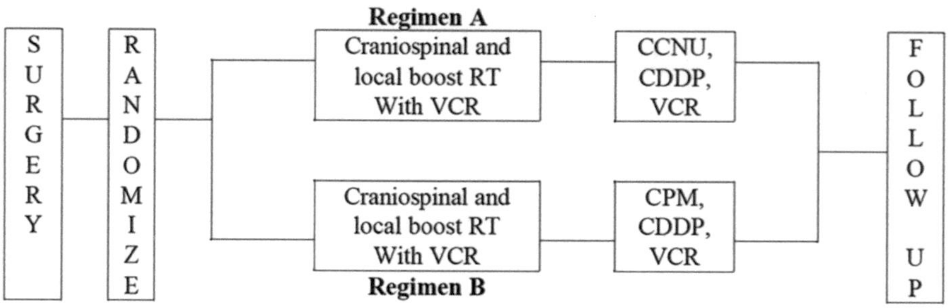

Figure 1.
Protocol A9961 treatment schematic [14].

The study gave us insight into developing strategies to manage clinical trials to make certain the requirements of the study and data management infrastructure can answer study questions including questions with chemotherapy. In retrospect, multiple patients were excluded from analysis as many had incomplete data including inability to assess post-surgery studies. The study was completed at a time when data were submitted through hard copy and courier; therefore, pre-treatment review of imaging and RT objects could not be performed. Because two cooperative groups were involved in the study (both later merged together as the COG), on-treatment review of objects was mandated for the POG institutions and not for CCG institutions as on-treatment review of imaging and RT objects was not an established component of the CCG data management process. The study foreshadowed the need for process improvements in clinical trial data management if the trial was going to be successful. Upon retrospective review of available imaging objects, more than 10% of the study patients had image-guided evidence of high-risk disease including a larger tumor burden of 1.5 cm^2 in the posterior fossa and/or disseminated disease in the cerebral spinal pathways. In the study, survival was only 36% in this subgroup of patients. Because half of the patient population had radiation oncology objects reviewed in a retrospective manner, there was a considerable number of treatment volume major study deviations largely centered on coverage of the cribriform plate, skull base, and posterior fossa boost. Interestingly, unlike other similar studies, the deviations in this study did not uniformly affect the study outcome upon review, particularly in the posterior fossa. This likely influenced the structure of COG ACNS0331, which sought to evaluate the use of an image-guided boost to the surgical cavity and not intentionally include the entire contents of the posterior fossa as in A9961 [16]. The assumption was if exclusion of segments of the anatomically defined posterior fossa were unintentionally excluded in the RT treatment field and did not directly affect local control or study outcome, perhaps a titrated volume directed to an image-guided disease target would be sufficient for protocol and clinical care management for patients with this disease [15].

The study also pointed out the importance of imaging in clinical trials and the application of imaging to the field of radiation oncology. If images were made available for central review prior to initiation of therapy coupled with the review for response assessment and pattern of failure, the number of ineligible patients on this study would have been significantly decreased and the study would potentially be powered to answer additional study questions. If patients are not treated to radiation volumes that are study compliant and less than the protocol dose is delivered to therapy targets, it becomes daunting to assess the success of chemotherapy. Each component of a trial plays an important role, and each treatment, response assessment, and pathology validation becomes essential to the mission if the results of the study are to be trusted and applied to clinical care. This study provided direction for how trials need to be managed to generate validation of the process and outcome. Imaging is our best tool to find common ground between investigators and institutions who participate in clinical trials, and it serves to support the effectiveness of chemotherapy in a quantitative manner [15].

3.2 ACNS0332

This MB study was designed to address the effectiveness of chemotherapy intensification with carboplatin used as a sensitizer to RT and isotretinoin as a proapoptotic therapeutic agent in patients with high-risk MB coupled with correlative biology studies. High-risk features included metastasis, residual disease, and diffuse anaplasia on pathology. This population received 36 Gy RT to the craniospinal axis with weekly VCR with/without carboplatin followed by six cycles of maintenance chemotherapy using CDDP, VCR, and CPM with/without 12 cycles of isotretinoin during and following maintenance chemotherapy (**Figure 2**). This study was important as it supported distinctions in response to therapy with biomarker analysis and opened the door to alternate approaches to chemotherapy and RT to molecular subgroups within the MB patient population [17, 18]. During the conduct of ACNS0332, four molecular subtypes of medulloblastoma were defined, namely Wingless-type mouse mammary tumor virus integration site (WNT), Sonic Hedgehog (SHH), Group 3, and Group 4 [17].

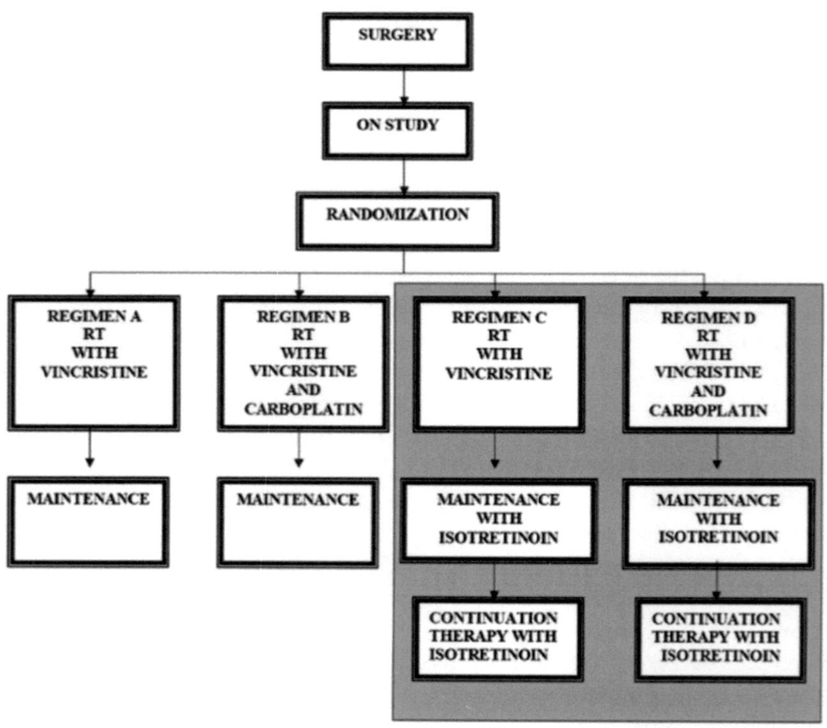

Figure 2.
Protocol ACNS0332 treatment schematic.

The isotretinoin component of the study was closed early due to futility; however, there was a significant 19% advantage at 5 years for the Group 3 patients receiving carboplatin supporting the use of intensification treatment strategies in this high-risk patient population. For this high-risk population, the 5-year disease-free survival was 66.4%. Of importance in this study was the identification that tumors that were part of the WNT (wingless and proto-oncogene Int1) pathway-activated biomarker demonstrated 100% 5-year survival, with the SHH biomarker disease demonstrating 53.6% 5-year survival, Group 3 demonstrating 73.7% 5-year survival, and Group 4 demonstrating 76.9% 5-year survival. Overall survival and EFS at 5 years in all groups were 73.4% and 62.9%, respectively [18].

3.3 ACNS0331

More studies continue to be done to evaluate the efficacy of lower CSRT doses with increased chemotherapy doses. One study did this by increasing chemotherapy doses using anti-leptomeningeal drugs while lowering the boost volume dose (focused dose to the area of the tumor bed plus an additional circumscribed margin, rather than treating the entire posterior fossa). Patients aged 3–7 were randomized to reduced-dose CSRT (18 Gy) or standard-dose CSRT and were then randomized to smaller-volume boost (RT to tumor bed +5.4 Gy to posterior fossa) or standard-volume boost. Patients received adjuvant VCR during RT. Patients then received maintenance chemotherapy for nine cycles, which followed an AAB cycling pattern. Therapy A is CDDP, CCNU, and VCR, and Therapy B is CPM, VCR, and mesna. Patients aged 8–21 received standard-dose CSRT and were then randomized to smaller-volume boost or standard-volume boost, with adjuvant VCR, followed by the same maintenance therapy (**Figure 3**) [16].

This was a study of considerable importance to the field of MB therapy. The study asked important questions of the RT community and, in turn, addressed issues

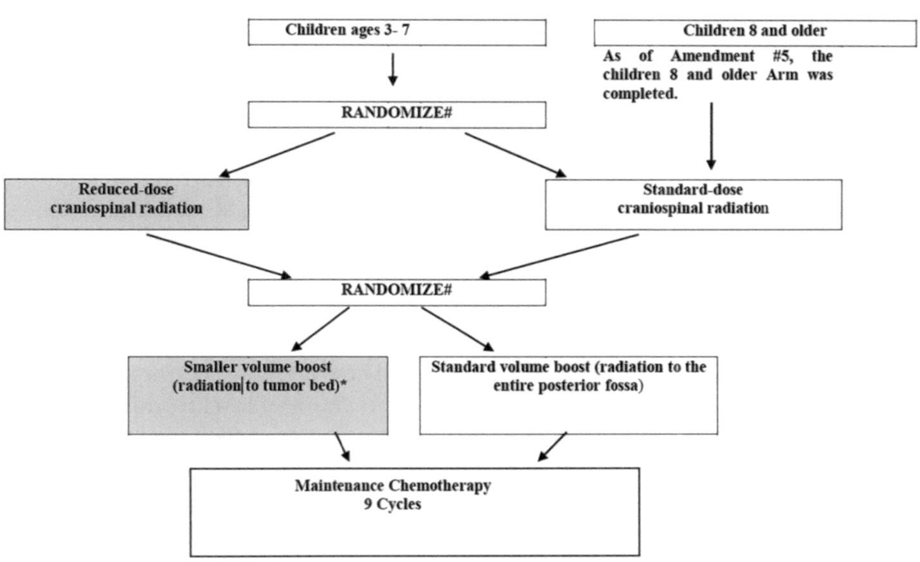

Figure 3.
ACNS0331 treatment schematic.

associated with integration of chemotherapy with alterations in RT. Prior to the development of advanced technology volumetric imaging, the radiation oncology community used anatomic guidelines to treat the posterior fossa as part of a boost or final-phase strategy after completion of cranial spinal RT. In this study, patients had an imbedded randomization to receiving final-phase RT to the traditional target volume or the image-guided surgical cavity defined by the postoperative surgical cavity with consideration to include potential tissues at risk defined on pre-operative imaging. This was made possible because of the advent of volumetric magnetic resonance imaging coupled with process improvements in digital data transfer tools permitting rapid acquisition of data and pre-therapy review of objects at quality assurance centers. The RT treatment objects were reviewed in real time with pre-therapy feedback given to sites for adjustments in the plan if needed to ensure RT compliance to protocol guidelines. Therefore, the execution of RT on study was highly consistent with study objectives relative to target volumes and radiation dose and confirmed that volume-specific RT targets were not inferior to traditional posterior fossa treatment volumes. The study also asked an important question as to whether radiation dose to the craniospinal axis could be reduced in patients seven or younger in order to limit toxicity imposed by therapy. The study demonstrated that dose reduction for younger children was not feasible for the general population. However, due to the suggestion in other studies that select subgroups of patients have excellent outcomes with titrated therapy, there may be an opportunity to revisit RT dose titration in patients with established favorable prognosis.

3.4 Current trials

One of the challenges in performing clinical trials in selected subgroups in MB is meeting accrual objectives to study important questions within the subgroups. In this disease, there are a limited number of patients within the subgroups, and most trials have studied the subsets as part of a larger trial treating all patients in a uniform manner evaluating response within the subset. A recent protocol was designed in COG to devise an alternate care strategy to MB patients with the favorable WNT biomarker. WNT expression comprises 10% of the MB population. The goal is to study patients >3 years and <22 years with this expression product and who have standard risk features including negative cerebral spinal fluid and <1.5 cm^2 residual disease in the posterior fossa. The protocol uses a reduced-dose cranial spinal therapy (18 Gy) with a boost to the image-guided target (36 Gy) for a total dose of 54 Gy. Unlike most protocols, the patients on study do not receive vincristine VCR during RT. Maintenance chemotherapy is delivered at a limited dose in alternating A and B cycles. Cycle A includes CDDP (75 mg/m^2), CCNU (75 mg/m^2 oral dose), and VCR (1.5 mg/m^2) on day 1 and VCR (1.5 mg/m^2) on days 8 and 15. Cycle B includes CPM (1000 mg/m^2-days 1 and 2) and VCR and mesna with CPM [19].

The study titrates both RT and chemotherapy. The study has been activated, and the results will help evaluate the ability to titrate therapy to a favorable patient population and conduct a trial in a subgroup of patients with MB. This is important for clinical trials in this disease. As biomarker-associated therapies become more available for management of subgroups of patients affected with this disease, it will be important to establish protocol driven pathways as both individual and integrated pathways to make clinical translational progress in this disease.

Likewise, an additional current study seeks to evaluate the efficacy of sodium thiosulfate during CDDP-containing chemotherapy cycles in reducing ototoxicity in children with average-risk MB. One such study seeks to evaluate whether sodium thiosulfate treatment will reduce this toxicity and not negatively influence outcome. The average-risk cohort receives 23.4 Gy CSI and 30.6 Gy IFRT boost, while the low-risk cohort receives 18 Gy CSI and 36 Gy involved-field RT (IFRT) boost. Risk is based on molecular and karyotype profiling. Maintenance chemotherapy is given for nine cycles in an AAB cycling pattern, with Cycle A containing CDDP, CCNU, VCR, and sodium thiosulfate (12.8 g/m^2 at day 1), whereas Cycle B contains cyclophosphamide, mesna, and vincristine. The use of cavity-targeted RT will also help address issues associated with ototoxicity [20].

The protocols have matured over several decades, and each was built on strong science available at the time of the development of the study. In diseases such as MB, one of the challenges is meeting accrual goals to ensure the study is powered to meet the objectives of the study. For protocol A9961, 189 institutions were required to participate in the study to meet the accrual objective of 421 patients [21]. Therefore, trial guidelines need to be written in a manner to encourage worldwide participation. In turn, this requires that the quality assurance program and data management platforms be strong with the ability to provide feedback to sites and site investigators in real (same day) time to ensure the quality of the data and plan compliance to study objectives including validation that the correct patient has been enrolled in the correct study. As many as 10% of patients were found ineligible for study, largely due to upstaging patients to high-risk status following retrospective review of pre-study imaging, which upon review demonstrated evidence of disease in the spine and greater than 1.5 cm^2 residual disease in the posterior fossa. Improved quality assurance programs including real-time study review by study investigators supporting onsite investigators have greatly facilitated this process and have served the following protocols well as we begin to study subsets of medulloblastoma patients in clinical trials [11, 22].

4. Future vision

The classification of MB is both histological and genetic, and recent associations between the two may be the basis for future methods of treatment. Histologically, MB is classified into the classic, desmoplastic/nodular (DN), extensive nodularity (MBEN), large cell/anaplastic (LCA), and not-otherwise specified subtypes, with the classic variant being the most common (72% of all MBs) [15, 23–25]. These tumors are composed of normocytic cells with round nuclei with infrequent mitoses. Homer Wright rosettes are commonly seen [26, 27]. DN MB has areas of neurocytic differentiation with surrounding areas of embryonal character. These tumors also have collagen deposits around cells [28], which are detectable with reticulin staining. The MBs with extensive nodularity (MBEN) (variant of DN MB) are frequently found in infants and have more irregular nodules that merge [25]. The LCA MB is typically divided into large-cell and anaplastic subtypes. Anaplastic MB is marked histologically by larger, more pleiomorphic tumor cells with increased mitoses, prominent nucleoli, as well as apoptotic tumor cells, whereas the large-cell subtype has less pleiomorphism but maintains the high rate of mitosis and apoptosis [24, 29]. Since 2016, anaplastic and large-cell MBs have been combined into one histologic category, as the two are often difficult to distinguish from one another. The LCA MB is associated with worse prognosis/higher risk when compared with the classic subtype [29, 30].

Importantly, the histologic features of some MB subtypes were found to be correlated with certain molecular features, which may represent a future vision of more targeted therapies in MB. Specifically, desmoplastic/nodular MB was found to be associated with SHH-activated tumors. LCA MB is correlated with MYC and MYCN amplification, SHH tumors with TP53 variations, and the G3 molecular subtype [31]. While surgical resection, RT, and chemotherapy remain the mainstay of treatment in MB, current advances in MB include targeted molecular therapy based on these new biomarker/pathology correlates.

Recent advances have shown certain mutations correlate with certain subgroups of MB, providing more specific tumor classification. The WNT tumors were found to be associated with CTNNB1, TP53, DDX3X, MLL2/3 mutations, TNRC6C methylation, and OTX2 and CDK6 amplifications. Overall, the WNT molecular subgroup is associated with high 5-year survival (97% in WNT α and 100% in WNT β) [24, 31–33]; SHH tumors are associated with PTCH1, SMO, SUFU, TP53, DDX3X, CREBBP, MLL2/3, TERT, and KDM6A mutations; TNR6C6, MX11, and IL8 methylation; MYCN, CDK6, and GLI2 amplification; and PTEN loss [24, 31, 33]. SHH α and β have 69.8% and 67.3% 5-year survival, respectively. SHH γ and δ have higher 5-year survival, at 88% and 88.5%, respectively. Molecular subgroup 3 (Non-WNT/non-SHH) is associated with TERT and KDM6A mutations; TNRC6C, MX11, and IL8 methylation; MYC, OTX2, and CDK6 amplification; KDM6A loss; and KBTBD4 insertion. Group 3 is associated with worse prognosis and the highest metastatic potential, with 5-year survival of 66.2%, 55.8%, and 41.9% in subgroups 3α, 3β, and 3γ, respectively. Subgroup 3γ has the lowest 5-year survival of all subgroups [31, 34, 35], In addition, studies have found Group 3 MB pathogenesis to be regulated by PRUNE-1 amplification, with PRUNE-1 being regulated by LSD1/KDM1A [34, 36]. Lastly, Group 4 (non-WNT/non-SHH) is associated with TERT and KDM6A mutations; TNRC6C, MX11, and IL8 methylation; Lmx1A enhancer activation, PRDM6 induction; MYCN, OTX2, and CDK6 amplification; PTEN and KDM6A loss; and KBTBD4 insertion. Five-year survival is 66.8%, 75.4%, and 82.5% in the 4α, 4β, and 4γ subgroups, respectively [31, 35, 37].

Many MB tumors are associated with SHH activation, so current approaches to target this signaling pathways may prove beneficial. Vismodegib, sonidegib, and glasdegib are SMO inhibitors that may be effective on tumors with mutations in the SHH pathway; however, mutations downstream of SMO may not benefit from this treatment [31, 33, 38]. Phase I studies performed by LoRusso et al. and Gajjar et al. of vismodegib showed an acceptable safety profile [39, 40]. LoRusso et al. showed vismodegib had antitumor activity in 20/68 patients (including the one patient in the study with MB) [39, 40]. Gajjar et al. showed antitumor activity in 1 of 3 SHH-subtype MB patients [39]. Rodon et al. showed sonidegib was safe and had antitumor activity in 3/9 patients with MB [41]. Robinson et al. showed vismodegib was safe and had antitumor activity in 4/40 SHH-subgroup MB patients. Robinson et al. showed vismodegib may have antitumor effects in adults with recurrent SHH-MB in two phase II studies [42]. As stated, SMO inhibitors may only have efficacy for tumors with mutations upstream of SMO. In addition, GL1 transcription factors mediate the HH pathway, which is often activated alongside the SHH pathway in medulloblastoma [31, 38]. Glioma-associated oncogene antagonist-61 (GANT61) is a GL1 antagonist shown to cause apoptosis in MB tumor cells. Arsenic trioxide has also been shown to block GLI1 transcription, which may also prove beneficial in SHH-activated MB, but it is still being used in preclinical models [31, 38].

PI3K pathway modifications have also been proven to be implicated in MB pathogenesis. Novel methods to target this pathway include BEZ235 (PI3K inhibitor) combined with vismodegib, which may be a promising treatment strategy. Additionally, the PI3K inhibitor samotolisib is currently being used to treat MB in clinical trials [31].

Another future direction for WNT-MB is to target the WNT/β-catenin pathway with PRI-724, a CREBBP-CTNNB1-interacting antagonist; however, this is not currently being used to treat MB [31, 38, 43].

The CDK4/6 signaling pathway is also implicated in non-WNT MBs, and targeting it has shown some success. Palbociclib (CDK4/6 inhibitor) has been shown to be effective in the Group 3 molecular subgroup and is being used in other trials for other subgroups [31, 38, 44]. Additionally, loading CDK4/6 inhibitors on nanoparticles may increase delivery of drug to tumor tissues. This is currently being tested in mouse models [45].

As Group 3 MB is mediated by PRUNE-1 and LSD1/KDM1A, novel approaches targeting these pathways represent hope in treating this subtype given its poor prognosis [34, 36]. A study done by Bibbò et al. showed that the combination of a PRUNE-1 inhibitor (AA7.1) and a LSD1/KDM1A inhibitor (SP-2577) inhibited tumor cytotoxicity, down-regulated N-cadherin expression, and inhibited tumor oxidative phosphorylation through altered mitochondrial metabolism [34].

Lastly, MYC-pathway disruptors, like JQ1 and BRD4 (bromodomain inhibitor) are thought to be another strategy in treating MYC-activated tumors, which are associated with poor prognosis and Group 3 MB; however, this therapy is not currently being tested [31, 46]. SETD8 inhibitors may also target this pathway by targeting the chromatin in genes implicated in MYC-mutated tumors [38, 47].

Other therapeutic approaches that researchers are considering are the development of targeted miRNAs associated with certain subgroups, as well as other molecular mutations that are highly associated with MB including DDX3x [30]. One small molecule inhibitor of DDX3 is RK-33, which has shown promise in causing cell cycle arrest and decreased expression downstream genes in the MB-WNT pathway [48].

5. Conclusions

Considerable progress has been made over the past decades incorporating chemotherapy regimens into the care of patients with medulloblastoma, both as agents to improve outcome and likewise balance the sequelae imposed by radiation management and provide patients with the better of both worlds. With the advent and use of molecular biology classification of disease, future treatment strategies will include targeted agents associated with biomarkers, which may both further promote the use of systemic therapy in this disease and titrate the use of traditional chemotherapy. We are at the edge of a new age in this disease, and it is likely not long before the paradigm will shift toward target-specific therapies as part of systemic therapy in this disease. While traditional treatment has had success, change is evident, and patients will benefit.

Acknowledgements

The Children's Oncology Group is supported by the National Institutes of Health (U10CA180886, U10CA180899) and the St. Baldrick's Foundation.

Conflict of interest

The authors declare no conflict of interest.

Author details

Julia Hayden[1], Stefanie Lowas[2,3], Nura El-Haj[2,3], Naheed Usmani[3], Koren Smith[1], Matthew Iandoli[1], Fran Laurie[1], Maryann Bishop-Jodoin[1], Eric Ko[1,4] and Paul Rava[1,4]*

1 Department Radiation Oncology, University of Massachusetts Chan Medical School, Worcester, MA, USA

2 Department of Pediatrics, University of Massachusetts Chan Medical School, Worcester, MA, USA

3 Department of Pediatrics, University of Massachusetts Health Care with UMass Memorial Health, Worcester, MA, USA

4 Department Radiation Oncology, University of Massachusetts Health Care with UMass Memorial Health, Worcester, MA, USA

*Address all correspondence to: paul.rava2@umassmed.edu

References

[1] Dressler EV, Dolecek TA, Liu M, Villano JL. Demographics, patterns of care, and survival in pediatric medulloblastoma. Journal of Neuro-Oncology. 2017;**132**(3):497-506. DOI: 10.1007/s11060-017-2400-5

[2] Seidel C, Heider S, Hau P, Glasow A, Dietzsch S, Kortmann RD. Radiotherapy in medulloblastoma—Evolution of treatment, current concepts and future perspectives. Cancers (Basel). 2021;**13**(23):5945. DOI: 10.3390/cancers13235945

[3] Armstrong GT, Jain N, Liu W, Merchant TE, Stovall M, Srivastava DK, et al. Region-specific radiotherapy and neuropsychological outcomes in adult survivors of childhood CNS malignancies. Neuro-Oncology. 2010;**12**(11):1173-1186. DOI: 10.1093/neuonc/noq104

[4] Christopherson KM, Rotondo RL, Bradley JA, Pincus DW, Wynn TT, Fort JA, et al. Late toxicity following craniospinal radiation for early-stage medulloblastoma. Acta Oncologica. 2014;**53**(4):471-480. DOI: 10.3109/0284186X.2013.862596

[5] Mulhern RK, Palmer SL, Merchant TE, Wallace D, Kocak M, Brouwers P, et al. Neurocognitive consequences of risk-adapted therapy for childhood medulloblastoma. Journal of Clinical Oncology. 2005;**23**(24):5511-5519. DOI: 10.1200/JCO.2005.00.703

[6] Xu W, Janss A, Packer RJ, Phillips P, Goldwein J, Moshang T Jr. Endocrine outcome in children with medulloblastoma treated with 18 Gy of craniospinal radiation therapy. Neuro-Oncology. 2004;**6**(2):113-118. DOI: 10.1215/s1152851703000462

[7] Balasubramanian S, Shobana MK. Pediatric craniospinal irradiation—The implementation and use of normal tissue complication probability in comparing photon versus proton planning. Journal of Medical Physics. 2021;**46**(4):244-252. DOI: 10.4103/jmp.jmp_75_21

[8] Phi JH, Lee J, Wang KC, Cho BK, Kim IO, Park CK, et al. Cerebrospinal fluid M staging for medulloblastoma: Reappraisal of Chang's M staging based on the CSF flow. Neuro-Oncology. 2011;**13**(3):334-344. DOI: 10.1093/neuonc/noq171

[9] Hartley KA, Li C, Laningham FH, Krasin MJ, Xiong X, Merchant TE. Vertebral body growth after craniospinal irradiation. International Journal of Radiation Oncology, Biology, Physics. 2008;**70**(5):1343-1349. DOI: 10.1016/j.ijrobp.2007.08.085

[10] Michiels EM, Schouten-Van Meeteren AY, Doz F, Janssens GO, van Dalen EC. Chemotherapy for children with medulloblastoma. Cochrane Database of Systematic Reviews. 2015;**1**(1):CD006678. DOI: 10.1002/14651858.CD006678

[11] FitzGerald TJ, Bishop-Jodoin M, Laurie F, Iandoli M, Smith K, Ulin K, et al. The importance of quality assurance in radiation oncology clinical trials. Seminars in Radiation Oncology. 2023;**33**(4):395-406. DOI: 10.1016/j.semradonc.2023.06.005

[12] Kalapurakal JA, Wolden SL, Haas-Kogan D, Laack NN, Hua CH, Paulino AC, et al. Children's Oncology Group's 2023 blueprint for research: Radiation oncology. Pediatric Blood & Cancer. 2023;**70**(Suppl. 6):e30593. DOI: 10.1002/pbc.30593

[13] Smith K, Ulin K, Knopp M, Kry S, Xiao Y, Rosen M, et al. Quality improvements in radiation oncology clinical trials. Frontiers in Oncology. 2023;**13**:1015596. DOI: 10.3389/fonc.2023.1015596

[14] Packer RJ, Zhou T, Holmes E, Vezina G, Gajjar A. Survival and secondary tumors in children with medulloblastoma receiving radiotherapy and adjuvant chemotherapy: Results of Children's Oncology Group trial A9961. Neuro-Oncology. 2013;**15**(1):97-103. DOI: 10.1093/neuonc/nos267

[15] Packer RJ, Gajjar A, Vezina G, Rorke-Adams L, Burger PC, Robertson PL, et al. Phase III study of craniospinal radiation therapy followed by adjuvant chemotherapy for newly diagnosed average-risk medulloblastoma. Journal of Clinical Oncology. 2006;**24**(25):4202-4208. DOI: 10.1200/JCO.2006.06.4980

[16] Michalski JM, Janss AJ, Vezina LG, Smith KS, Billups CA, Burger PC, et al. Children's Oncology Group Phase III trial of reduced-dose and reduced-volume radiotherapy with chemotherapy for newly diagnosed average-risk medulloblastoma. Journal of Clinical Oncology. 2021;**39**(24):2685-2697. DOI: 10.1200/JCO.20.02730

[17] Chemotherapy and Radiation Therapy in Treating Young Patients With Newly Diagnosed, Previously Untreated, High-Risk Medulloblastoma//PNET [Internet]. 2024. Available from: https://clinicaltrials.gov/study/NCT00392327 [Accessed: April 12, 2024]

[18] Leary SES, Packer RJ, Li Y, Billups CA, Smith KS, Jaju A, et al. Efficacy of carboplatin and isotretinoin in children with high-risk medulloblastoma: A randomized clinical trial from the children's oncology group. JAMA Oncology. 2021;**7**(9):1313-1321. DOI: 10.1001/jamaoncol.2021.2224

[19] Patel S, Alam A, Pant R, Chattopadhyay S. Wnt signaling and its significance within the tumor microenvironment: Novel therapeutic insights. Frontiers in Immunology. 2019;**10**:2872. DOI: 10.3389/fimmu.2019.02872

[20] Knight KR, Kraemer DF, Neuwelt EA. Ototoxicity in children receiving platinum chemotherapy: Underestimating a commonly occurring toxicity that may influence academic and social development. Journal of Clinical Oncology. 2005;**23**(34):8588-8596. DOI: 10.1200/JCO.2004.00.5355

[21] FitzGerald TJ, Followill D, Laurie F, Boterberg T, Hanusik R, Kessel S, et al. Quality assurance in radiation oncology. Pediatric Blood & Cancer. 2021;**68**(Suppl. 2):e28609. DOI: 10.1002/pbc.28609

[22] Donahue B, Marymont MA, Kessel S, Iandoli MK, Fitzgerald T, Holmes E, et al. Radiation therapy quality in CCG/POG intergroup 9961: Implications for craniospinal irradiation and the posterior fossa boost in future medulloblastoma trials. Frontiers in Oncology. 2012;**2**:185. DOI: 10.3389/fonc.2012.00185

[23] Ellison D. Classifying the medulloblastoma: Insights from morphology and molecular genetics. Neuropathology and Applied Neurobiology. 2002;**28**(4):257-282. DOI: 10.1046/j.1365-2990.2002.00419.x

[24] Ellison DW, Dalton J, Kocak M, Nicholson SL, Fraga C, Neale G, et al. Medulloblastoma: Clinicopathological correlates of SHH, WNT, and non-SHH/WNT molecular subgroups. Acta Neuropathologica. 2011;**121**(3):381-396. DOI: 10.1007/s00401-011-0800-8

[25] McManamy CS, Pears J, Weston CL, Hanzely Z, Ironside JW, Taylor RE, et al. Nodule formation and desmoplasia in medulloblastomas-defining the nodular/desmoplastic variant and its biological behavior. Brain Pathology. 2007;**17**(2):151-164. DOI: 10.1111/j.1750-3639.2007.00058.x

[26] Burger PC, Grahmann FC, Bliestle A, Kleihues P. Differentiation in the medulloblastoma. A histological and immunohistochemical study. Acta Neuropathologica. 1987;**73**(2):115-123. DOI: 10.1007/BF00693776

[27] Wippold FJ 2nd, Perry A. Neuropathology for the neuroradiologist: Rosettes and pseudorosettes. AJNR. American Journal of Neuroradiology. 2006;**27**(3):488-492

[28] Rodriguez FJ, Eberhart C, O'Neill BP, Slezak J, Burger PC, Goldthwaite P, et al. Histopathologic grading of adult medulloblastomas. Cancer. 2007;**109**(12):2557-2565. DOI: 10.1002/cncr.22717

[29] Orr BA. Pathology, diagnostics, and classification of medulloblastoma. Brain Pathology. 2020;**30**(3):664-678. DOI: 10.1111/bpa.12837

[30] Ramaswamy V, Remke M, Bouffet E, Bailey S, Clifford SC, Doz F, et al. Risk stratification of childhood medulloblastoma in the molecular era: The current consensus. Acta Neuropathologica. 2016;**131**(6):821-831. DOI: 10.1007/s00401-016-1569-6

[31] Zhou Z, Zhu B, Meng Q, Zhang T, Wu Y, Yu R, et al. Research progress in molecular pathology markers in medulloblastoma. Exploration of Targeted Anti-tumor Therapy. 2023;**4**(1):139-156. DOI: 10.37349/etat.2023.00126

[32] Clifford SC, Lusher ME, Lindsey JC, Langdon JA, Gilbertson RJ, Straughton D, et al. Wnt/Wingless pathway activation and chromosome 6 loss characterize a distinct molecular sub-group of medulloblastomas associated with a favorable prognosis. Cell Cycle. 2006;**5**(22):2666-2670. DOI: 10.4161/cc.5.22.3446

[33] Kool M, Jones DT, Jäger N, Northcott PA, Pugh TJ, Hovestadt V, et al. Genome sequencing of SHH medulloblastoma predicts genotype-related response to smoothened inhibition. Cancer Cell. 2014;**25**(3): 393-405. DOI: 10.1016/j.ccr.2014.02.004

[34] Bibbò F, Asadzadeh F, Boccia A, Sorice C, Bianco O, Saccà CD, et al. Targeting group 3 medulloblastoma by the anti-PRUNE-1 and anti-LSD1/KDM1A epigenetic molecules. International Journal of Molecular Sciences. 2024;**25**(7):3917. DOI: 10.3390/ijms25073917

[35] Brandes AA, Bartolotti M, Marucci G, Ghimenton C, Agati R, Fioravanti A, et al. New perspectives in the treatment of adult medulloblastoma in the era of molecular oncology. Critical Reviews in Oncology/Hematology. 2015;**94**(3):348-359. DOI: 10.1016/j.critrevonc.2014.12.016

[36] Ferrucci V, de Antonellis P, Pennino FP, Asadzadeh F, Virgilio A, Montanaro D, et al. Metastatic group 3 medulloblastoma is driven by PRUNE1 targeting NME1-TGF-β-OTX2-SNAIL via PTEN inhibition. Brain. 2018;**141**(5):1300-1319. DOI: 10.1093/brain/awy039

[37] Jones DT, Jäger N, Kool M, Zichner T, Hutter B, Sultan M, et al. Dissecting the genomic complexity underlying medulloblastoma. Nature. 2012;**488**(7409):100-105. DOI: 10.1038/nature11284

[38] Gatto L, Franceschi E, Tosoni A, Di Nunno V, Bartolini S, Brandes AA.

Molecular targeted therapies: Time for a paradigm shift in medulloblastoma treatment? Cancers (Basel). 2022;**14**(2):333. DOI: 10.3390/cancers14020333

[39] Gajjar A, Stewart CF, Ellison DW, Kaste S, Kun LE, Packer RJ, et al. Phase I study of vismodegib in children with recurrent or refractory medulloblastoma: A pediatric brain tumor consortium study. Clinical Cancer Research. 2013;**19**(22):6305-6312. DOI: 10.1158/1078-0432.CCR-13-1425

[40] LoRusso PM, Rudin CM, Reddy JC, Tibes R, Weiss GJ, Borad MJ, et al. Phase I trial of hedgehog pathway inhibitor vismodegib (GDC-0449) in patients with refractory, locally advanced or metastatic solid tumors. Clinical Cancer Research. 2011;**17**(8):2502-2511. DOI: 10.1158/1078-0432.CCR-10-2745

[41] Rodon J, Tawbi HA, Thomas AL, Stoller RG, Turtschi CP, Baselga J, et al. A phase I, multicenter, open-label, first-in-human, dose-escalation study of the oral smoothened inhibitor Sonidegib (LDE225) in patients with advanced solid tumors. Clinical Cancer Research. 2014;**20**(7):1900-1909. DOI: 10.1158/1078-0432.CCR-13-1710

[42] Robinson GW, Orr BA, Wu G, Gururangan S, Lin T, Qaddoumi I, et al. Vismodegib exerts targeted efficacy against recurrent Sonic Hedgehog-Subgroup medulloblastoma: Results from Phase II Pediatric Brain Tumor Consortium Studies PBTC-025B and PBTC-032. Journal of Clinical Oncology. 2015;**33**(24):2646-2654. DOI: 10.1200/JCO.2014.60.1591

[43] Fattet S, Haberler C, Legoix P, Varlet P, Lellouch-Tubiana A, Lair S, et al. Beta-catenin status in paediatric medulloblastomas: Correlation of immunohistochemical expression with mutational status, genetic profiles, and clinical characteristics. The Journal of Pathology. 2009;**218**(1):86-94. DOI: 10.1002/path.2514

[44] Cook Sangar ML, Genovesi LA, Nakamoto MW, Davis MJ, Knobluagh SE, Ji P, et al. Inhibition of CDK4/6 by Palbociclib significantly extends survival in medulloblastoma patient-derived xenograft mouse models. Clinical Cancer Research. 2017;**23**(19):5802-5813. DOI: 10.1158/1078-0432.CCR-16-2943

[45] Lim C, Dismuke T, Malawsky D, Ramsey JD, Hwang D, Godfrey VL, et al. Enhancing CDK4/6 inhibitor therapy for medulloblastoma using nanoparticle delivery and scRNA-seq-guided combination with sapanisertib. Science Advances. 2022;**8**(4):eabl5838. DOI: 10.1126/sciadv.abl5838

[46] Bandopadhayay P, Bergthold G, Nguyen B, Schubert S, Gholamin S, Tang Y, et al. BET bromodomain inhibition of MYC-amplified medulloblastoma. Clinical Cancer Research. 2014;**20**(4):912-925. DOI: 10.1158/1078-0432.CCR-13-2281

[47] Veo B, Danis E, Pierce A, Sola I, Wang D, Foreman NK, et al. Combined functional genomic and chemical screens identify SETD8 as a therapeutic target in MYC-driven medulloblastoma. JCI Insight. 2019;**4**(1):e122933. DOI: 10.1172/jci.insight.122933

[48] Tantravedi S, Vesuna F, Winnard PT Jr, Martin A, Lim M, et al. Targeting DDX3 in medulloblastoma using the small molecule inhibitor RK-33. Translational Oncology. 2019;**12**(1):96-105. DOI: 10.1016/j.tranon.2018.09.002

Chapter 5

Radiation Therapy for Medulloblastoma

David Harris, Jessica Yancey, Gavin Jones, Koren Smith, Sandy Kessel, Fran Laurie, Matthew Iandoli, Maryann Bishop-Jodoin, Yansong Geng, Linda Ding, Julie Trifone, Julia Hayden, Eric Ko and Paul Rava

Abstract

Radiation therapy remains a cornerstone in the clinical care of patients with medulloblastoma. Nevertheless, while treatment with radiation improves disease control, it is also associated with potential late effects impacting neurologic and neurocognitive function, pituitary function as well as hearing. The development of secondary, treatment-related malignancies is an uncommon but possible late outcome. In this chapter, we review the role of radiation therapy in medulloblastoma, as well as changes in management that have resulted both from technological therapeutic advancements and enterprising cooperative group clinical trials for this disease. Moreover, with increasing utilization of molecular diagnostics both for prognosis and stratification of treatment, we also endeavor to explore opportunities to further improve the delivery of radiation therapy to patients with varied risk of disease recurrence.

Keywords: radiation treatment, clinical trials, medulloblastoma, children, precision therapy

1. Introduction

Radiation therapy has played an important role in the management of patients with medulloblastoma. Historically, it was well-recognized from autopsy studies that medulloblastoma exhibited a propensity to spread through the ventricular pathways of the central nervous system (CNS). Investigators therefore acknowledged that radiation treatment volumes would necessarily need to include the entire neuroaxis and meningeal surface as part of a composite care plan, with treatment delivered to all potential sites of disease in a continuous manner on a daily basis. Likewise, because the tumor had access to fluid pathways at all time points of management, radiation oncology plans were designed to treat the meningeal surface during each treatment session. To these ends, additional dosimetric and treatment delivery strategies were employed to match radiation treatment fields while minimizing potential overlap of dose in critical normal tissue, the most significant of these being the spinal cord. These strategies generated success in tumor control. However, the epidemiology of medulloblastoma is such that more than 40% of patients affected with this disease are identified before the age of 5 and approximately 70% of patients affected by the disease are identified before the age of 10, a critical period of anatomical development in which important structures in the CNS, vertebral bodies, and other vulnerable normal tissue have not yet reached full maturity. Moreover, multiple additional normal tissues received collateral exit doses from spinal treatment fields, including but not limited to the posterior pharyngeal wall, thyroid, cardiopulmonary structures, small bowel, kidneys, and soft tissue pelvic structures. The vertebral bodies and pelvis bony structures were likewise at risk for injury and titration of growth and development, again visibly affecting the most vulnerable and youngest of the patients relative to both standing and sitting height. Modern clinical protocols work to address these issues through comprehensive review of outcomes and adjustments in therapy to attempt to mitigate these potential side effects. Although titration adjustments in the posterior fossa boost volume have been adopted without concomitant compromise in disease control, subsequent attempts to titrate both volume and dose of the entire neuroaxis have been decidedly less successful. Therefore, considerable work needs to be completed through modern risk categorization to determine if there are distinct medulloblastoma patient subpopulations—that is, those with otherwise more favorable disease biology—where radiation dose volume titration may be reasonable to revisit and study through investigatory clinical trials. Conversely, it is equally important to identify potential high-risk population cohorts who may stand to benefit from augmented or intensified therapy. Interdigitation with chemotherapy brings both strength and consequence as well as strategies to make certain that patients are given the benefits of both therapies without unintended risk of injury [1–6].

In this chapter, we review the history of radiation therapy in the treatment of medulloblastoma aligned with the development of modern technology to optimize tumor control with decreased risk. We also review the future role of radiation therapy with modern classification of pathology and biomarker expression products in consideration of additional adjustments that may be made in treatment technique and patient stratification moving forward.

2. History of radiation therapy in medulloblastoma and the development of treatment technique

In 1930, the Neurosurgeon Harvey Cushing first reported surgical resection of medulloblastoma located in the posterior fossa and identified the challenges and limitations of favorable patient outcomes due to leptomeningeal spread of disease throughout the neuroaxis, which limited the success of primary surgery. Recognizing the need to treat the entire meningeal surface, Edith Paterson and RF Farr published a manuscript from Christie hospital and the Holt Radium Institute (Manchester, England) using orthovoltage therapy to treat the entire neuroaxis. These investigators reported on 27 patients treated from 1941 to 1950 with pathology validated by a single pathologist. The authors confirmed that care was taken to include the entire CNS and skull base in the therapy field with the inferior limit of the spine field at the second sacral vertebra corresponding to thecal sac termination. The patients were treated with a single posterior field, including the entire CNS, with patients lying in the prone position. Lead was used to limit the width of the spine fields. The investigators found an advantage in tilting the spine field at 20 degrees toward the head to achieve a more uniform dose distribution through the treatment field. The anterior component of the cranium had dose augmented by supplementary fields as it was recognized that a single posterior field of radiation would be insufficient to cover intracranial contents. The patients were treated AP-PA with shielding applied to the posterior field to accommodate dose received in that location from the initial posterior field. Optimal dose was thought to be 3500 rads over 5 weeks. Results from this investigation revealed a 65% survival rate for the entire population at 5 years, with a 54% survival for children only. Observations at 3 years post-treatment included one child with neurocognitive limitations (which also pre-dated therapy) and shortening of sitting height in children treated at ages below the age of 10 [7, 8].

As linear accelerator technology became available in both Europe and North America, a more comprehensive understanding of the geometry of radiation fields became visible and cranial-spinal radiation therapy techniques matured with evolving technology. Because radiation beams generated from linear accelerators expanded at a distance in a pyramidal distribution, treatment planning strategies were developed to accommodate this geometry. Simply abutting the cranium and spine fields would result in overlap over the spinal cord, providing a greater dose than prescribed and an increased risk for permanent neurologic injury. Patients were treated in the prone or supine position with prone treatments more commonly preferred by radiation oncologists for reproducibility of a match line. Supine treatment, however, was preferred by pediatric anesthesiologists to allow airway protection in younger children who required anesthesia for daily treatment. With the cranium treated with lateral fields, the table would be rotated to create a non-divergent field edge at the inferior field border in order to carefully match the spine field to the head field. The collimator of the cranial field was angled to match the divergence angle of the spine field with a separation of 1 cm in order to create a "cold" match point over the cervical spine (**Figure 1**). The match point would be moved each day with three separate positions. This technique was referred to as "feathering" in order to make certain that the "cold" under-dosed region was not always in the same anatomic area. Demonstrating department and investigator expertise in this and similar techniques was a benchmark requirement for participation in clinical trials for the Children's Oncology Group (COG). Clinical and computational expertise was needed to ensure patients were treated in a uniform manner on study in order for the results of the study to be trusted

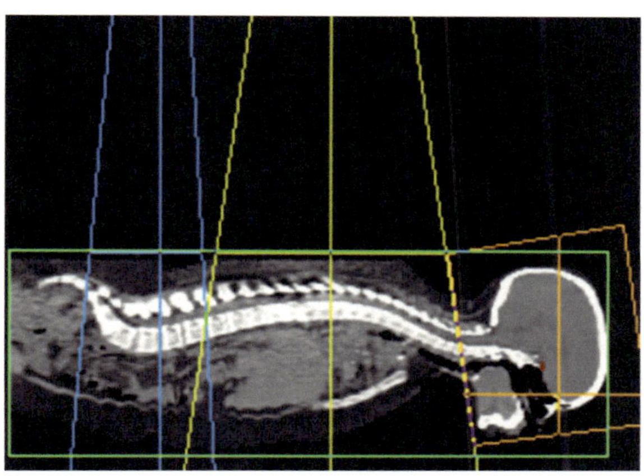

Figure 1.
Match fields over the cervical spine with the angle of the collimator of the cranial fields matching the divergence angle of the spine field. Field overlap in the lumbar region was deep to the cord ensuring absence of "hot spots" within this critical structure.

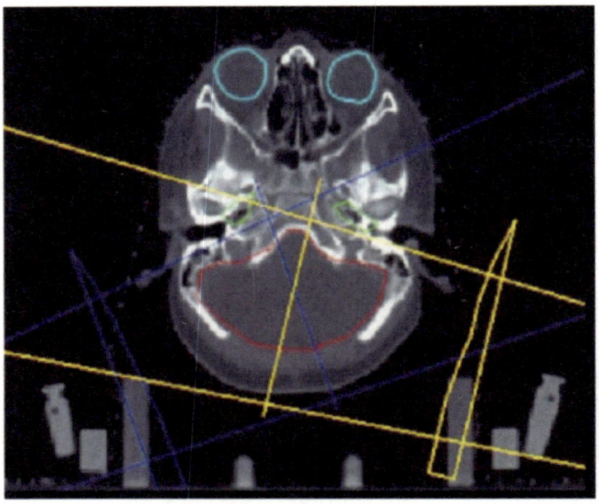

Figure 2.
Traditional boost fields generating prescription doses to the cochlea region.

and become incorporated into daily clinical management. These early investigator treatments were designed and delivered as two-dimensional field plans; however, with the emergence of volumetric and three-dimensional radiation therapy treatment planning tools, treatment execution would influence the approach to radiation therapy field design and drive planning toward disease associated and volumetric tumor targets [9–12].

One of the major challenges imposed by historical approaches to cranial-spinal radiation therapy is that the target of requisite CNS anatomy, including the entire meningeal surface, cribriform plate, skull base, and thecal sac—was covered by default, standard fields designated solely by two-dimensional planning. Often, deviations in medulloblastoma clinical protocols during this era were driven by incomplete coverage of these structures using two-dimensional geometry. Over-blocking of the orbits and skull base was generally the root cause of the study deviation and investigators could point toward recurrences of disease associated with incomplete anatomical coverage of targets. Boost strategies were also designed by clinical anatomical boundaries with the posterior fossa field design directed to the anterior clinoid, top of the tentorium, and internal occipital protuberance as targets (**Figure 2**). This generated increased consistency and treatment uniformity among investigators in radiation therapy field design; however, specific questions about dose titration to anatomical structures unintentionally treated including visual pathways, hippocampus, and cochlea could not be addressed through this mechanism as the dose received by normal tissue was equal to the prescription dose to the disease. As sequelae of management became more visible in outcome analysis, clinical trialists became interested in understanding quantitative volumetric dose. They investigated if conformal avoidance of normal tissue and dose volume titration of these structures could lessen toxicity [13–15].

3. Volumetric-based radiation oncology treatment planning for medulloblastoma

Treatment planning for radiation therapy moved from fluoroscopy to computed tomography (CT) with the advent of three-dimensional planning and forever changed the landscape for treatment planning in this disease. Individual structures within the CNS and spinal axis could be imaged, identified contoured as individual objects, with dose calculated to the volume of normal tissue. Investigators could now evaluate the relationship of dose to the clinical target and critical normal tissue in a developmental manner. For example, the cribriform plate resides in the same axial plane as the lens in children up until the approximate age of 9 years. At this time, the frontal sinus begins to mature, and by the age of 12, the cribriform plate is generally 1.2 cm superior and rostral to the lens. Therefore, if one over-blocked the orbit, the cribriform region would also be unintentionally blocked. Volumetric planning with CT reduced the likelihood of this error. In early clinical trials using volumetric imaging for the posterior fossa component of therapy, investigators could now visualize limitations in anatomically applied radiation therapy fields. Lateral fields would unintentionally include the cochlea to high dose, posterior fields would exit into the oral cavity, and vertex fields would exit into the thyroid delivering dose that would be unknowingly remarkably high in young children as the distance to the thyroid gland in a young child is much less than it is in an adult when viewed through the lens of a vertex field. Improving radiation field placement in these situations with field volume titration could be partially optimized through this process by extracting the best of each field while minimizing the negative consequence of each field. This process also established the importance of imaging in the evaluation of medulloblastoma.

Magnetic resonance imaging (MRI) with contrast has become the standard of care in this disease for both the spine and CNS. Staging, target definition, and follow-up care are all now influenced by this standard of care imaging; the presence and absence of residual disease in the posterior fossa, presence of spinal metastasis, location of the thecal sac, and oncologic treatment outcomes are all measured by imaging. Our neuroradiology colleagues are now integral members of the multidisciplinary treatment team.

Medulloblastoma protocol A9961 remains an excellent example of the importance of imaging and peer review of imaging on the study. Often, studies will identify criteria for measuring the presence or absence of residual disease and spinal metastasis, which may/may not coincide with specific institutional criteria. During a retrospective review of imaging on protocol A9961, approximately 10% of patients enrolled into the study were actually not study-eligible due to greater than 1.5 cm^2 residual tumor in the posterior fossa, or presence of spinal disease otherwise not identified at pre-study entry. An additional group of patients was ineligible due to the presence of motion artifact on submitted imaging, confounding the process of tumor quantification and disease assessment by designated study imaging reviewers. For this study, 189 institutions were needed to reach the accrual objective of 421 patients, therefore, the 10% loss in patient population was an unforeseen detriment for the assessment of this study outcome. Therefore, the quality of the imaging and its interpretation is an essential component of management of a successful study and the importance of imaging for these study patients cannot be overstated. Nevertheless, the protocol experience provided insight into how best to manage quality assurance of both imaging and radiation therapy in medulloblastoma. Additional issues with protocol execution were also revelatory and generative in the following manner: the protocol was an intergroup trial between the two pediatric clinical trial groups—the Children's Cancer Study Group (CCSG) and the Pediatric oncology Group (POG). CCSG, however, did not participate in pre-therapy review of treatment objects. As a result, there were multiple deviations on study, generally related to volume limitations at the level of the cribriform plate, skull base, and posterior fossa, thus limiting commensurate comparison of all patients as a singular cohort. This highlights one of the many challenges in clinical trial development and implementation: to create a uniform study population for the results of the trial to be trusted and translated directly into clinical practice [16–20].

By limiting study deviations with improvement in the rapid digital transfer of imaging and radiation therapy treatment objects to quality assurance centers, important questions in this disease could be answered with confidence that the quality and consistency of complex radiation delivery would not hinder the interpretation of the study. COG protocol ACNS0331 asked two important study questions related to radiation therapy. The central question was to evaluate whether the final phase of management had to be tailored to the anatomical configuration of the posterior fossa as historically described and performed. This study randomized the radiation posterior fossa boost to either historical anatomically defined fields or a more limited area of imaging-defined disease and the surgical cavity (involved field targeting). This change, if found valid, would, in turn, spare considerable normal tissue including the cochlea and temporal lobes from unnecessary radiation and late effects. ANCS0331 had quality assurance processes embedded in the trial to review imaging and radiation therapy treatment objects in real time to ensure the objects were of sufficient quality for study compliance and that the individual radiation therapy plans met protocol standards. The study successfully established involved field image guided targeting as the standard of care in these average risk patients for the final phase of management. The study also asked a question in patients 3–7 years of age as to whether or not the radiation dose in the first phase of craniospinal irradiation could be reduced to 18 Gy. This proved to be unsuccessful for the general population of medulloblastoma patients treated on this study. However, because of favorable outcomes for the 10% of medulloblastoma patients expressing Wingless-related integration site (WNT) biomarkers, an opportunity arose to revisit radiation dose titration and chemotherapy reduction in this distinct molecular subgroup of patients [21–24].

Newer protocols exclusively treating standard risk patients with WNT expression have embraced this task. Nevertheless, this is a challenging endeavor because the otherwise apparently favorable WNT biomarker is expressed in only around 10% of the entire medulloblastoma patient population; therefore, to effectively power the study, participation from centers worldwide is needed to meet accrual objectives. Because of the limited study population, the quality of data from each patient also needs to be complete and meet study objectives, as any deviation or limitation in data acquisition would hinder the goals and objectives of the study analysis. This likewise requires that the quality assurance centers have data management processes in situ that can respond to sites in real time, generally on a same-day basis for clinical trial management. The study will acquire valuable data to see if radiation and chemotherapy dose titration can be applied to a molecularly defined and favorable population. Because of nimble and effective data acquisition and transfer tools, prospective trials on limited subsets of patients can now be achieved with trusted outcomes [21].

4. The importance of imaging and how modern MRI signals influence staging

CNS MRI is the imaging modality of choice for the diagnosis of medulloblastoma. It aids in differentiating medulloblastoma from other pediatric CNS malignancies in addition to completing staging. Medulloblastoma classically presents on MRI as a midline posterior fossa tumor. The typical presentation of the tumor is hypo- or iso-intense on T1 images, heterogeneous or hypointense on T2, and enhancing on post-contrast T1 images [25, 26]. Diffusion-weighted imaging (DWI) and apparent diffusion coefficient (ADC) can aid in further differentiating medulloblastoma from other CNS tumors such as ependymomas and pilocytic astrocytomas [26, 27]. Risk stratification of medulloblastoma includes histological assessment, Chang staging, age, and amount of disease remaining post-operatively. MRI determines two of four risk stratification criteria. Chang staging is categorized as M0 through M4 and historically relied on CT and craniospinal fluid analysis. However, CT alone is typically unable to distinguish M0 from M2/3 disease (M2 is intracranial seeding, M3 is seeding in subarachnoid space), a distinction that could change a patient's risk stratification from low to high. MRI has replaced CT as its detailed diagnostics allow for the appreciation of gross seeding in the CNS [28]. In addition, post-operative brain MRI at 24–48 hours provides assessment of extent of resection and residual disease burden [27]. Greater than 1.5 cc^2 of residual disease is one of the components of high-risk disease [26, 29, 30]. Appropriate risk stratification is imperative to adjuvant treatment recommendations and therefore patient outcome.

Imaging has become an important adjudicator for both site and study investigators. Review of imaging in real time not only ensures correct staging but also allows for patients to be properly treated per protocol or randomized to the appropriate protocol. Because of real-time data management tools, trial investigators and radiologists worldwide have access to images on a same-day basis and can participate in management decisions in a timely manner. Investigators can in turn achieve consistency in the interpretation of both disease response and progression as well as making certain that patients assigned standard risk status by institutions are placed into the correct study. Imaging is essential to modern clinical trial management and is highly important to the quality assurance process for each trial.

5. The importance of molecular classification

In addition to clinically and imaging-defined risk stratification, molecular subtyping of medulloblastoma informs outcomes. Currently, there are four molecular subtypes of medulloblastoma: Group 3, Group 4, Sonic Hedgehog (SHH), and WNT [31, 32]. Although the determination of subtype is not currently incorporated into adjuvant treatment guidelines, there are groups actively investigating this question by integrating clinical and molecular risk-directed therapy approaches [31, 32]. Given that there can be limited accessibility to molecular testing, the interpretation of MRI for diagnosis of subtypes is also under investigation. One method to identify subtypes of medulloblastoma is based on generalized patterns of neuro-anatomic location. For example, Group 3/Group 4 tumors tend to arise in the 4th ventricle, whereas WNT tumors tend to arise within the Foramen of Luschka or adjacent cerebrospinal fluid spaces. However, it is important to remember that these correlations are not absolute. With advanced MRI sequences, further delineation of subtypes is becoming apparent based on the appearance on MRI images. Radiomics and machine learning algorithms are currently being used on presurgical MRIs to predict medulloblastoma subtypes. Zhang et al. found that T1-correlation is greater for SHH and lower for WNT. Reddy et al. found that Group 3/4 tumors showed the highest median ADC values in the enhancing sold tumor, in contrast with WNT tumors which had the lowest median ADC values [33]. MRI correlations to molecular subtypes will be further refined as protocol data matures and can be correlated to outcome imaging [28, 33, 34].

6. The importance of radiation therapy and quality assurance

The development of protocols in medulloblastoma foreshadowed the importance of imaging and quality assurance in the execution of radiation therapy in this disease. Investigators have recognized that study deviations in medulloblastoma treatment have the potential to influence individual patient outcomes. After deviations were identified in protocol A9961, study groups and investigators made efforts to build consensus in contouring objects in a standardized manner and create a uniform study group. Uniform study sets and patients with treatment executed in a protocol-compliant format become invaluable to investigators to study additional questions not anticipated at the time of trial design. Models can be developed to evaluate opportunities for improved patient care and generate metrics for toxicity evaluation during and after the study is completed [20, 22–24, 35–39].

Protocols also call attention to important steps forward for the management of medulloblastoma patients. Since the Paterson and Farr paper in 1953, radiation oncologists used the bony anatomy of the posterior fossa for the boost volume. This had convenience as the top of the tentorium was remarkably consistent at 7.5 cm from the top of the skull in an age-transparent fashion. Early radiation oncologists would place their thumb at the foramen magnum and extend the third finger to the top of the skull and the top of the tentorium would reside two-thirds distance from the foramen magnum. The posterior clinoid and the internal occipital protuberance would be the landmarks used to draw the "tent". The A9961 study evaluated the application of an image-guided boost directed to the surgical cavity as a point of randomization and the study demonstrated that volume titration was non-inferior to historical anatomical coverage. This was a major step forward for radiation oncology as we could now apply image-guided targeting to this disease and limit radiation dose to unintentional

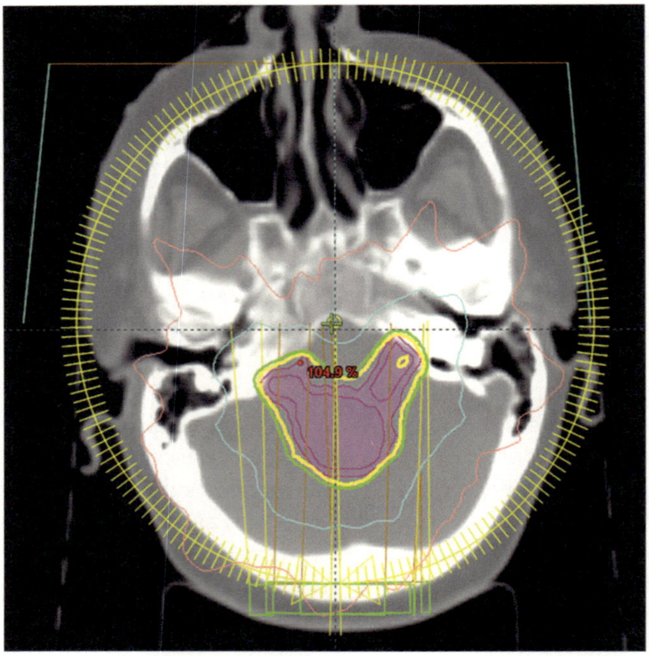

Figure 3.
Axial geometry of image guided boost using volumetric arcs generating minimal dose to the cochlea.

targets including but not limited to the cochlea and anterior brain stem in the proximity of the basilar artery. Because this was managed in a protocol setting, our discipline is confident in the outcome of the study, and this strategy for final phase management to an image-guided target sparing additional normal tissue has now been readily applied into standard clinical practice (**Figure 3**) [21].

The A9961 study also placed emphasis on developing consensus contouring anatomy for therapy. With fluoroscopic imaging, the cribriform plate and meningeal surface are at times challenging to visualize. If one contours what is seen as the brain/CNS, the egress points of cranial nerve exit through the skull will be under-contoured, and if not recognized, the meningeal surface would be unintentionally under-treated (**Figures 4** and **5**). When changes in practice habits occur and are

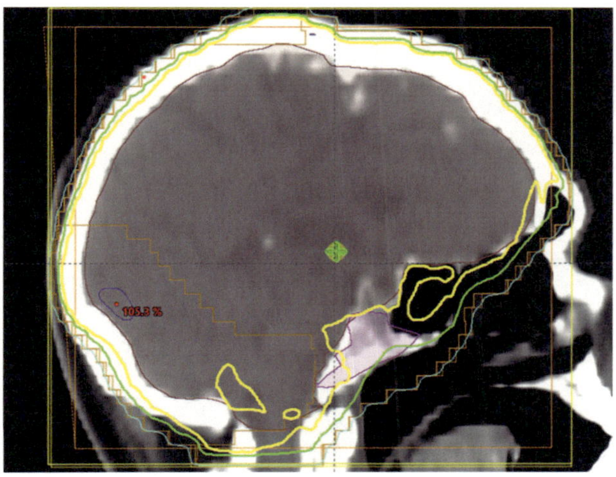

Figure 4.
Meningeal surface dose when targets are contoured through the clivus and egress points of the cranial nerves.

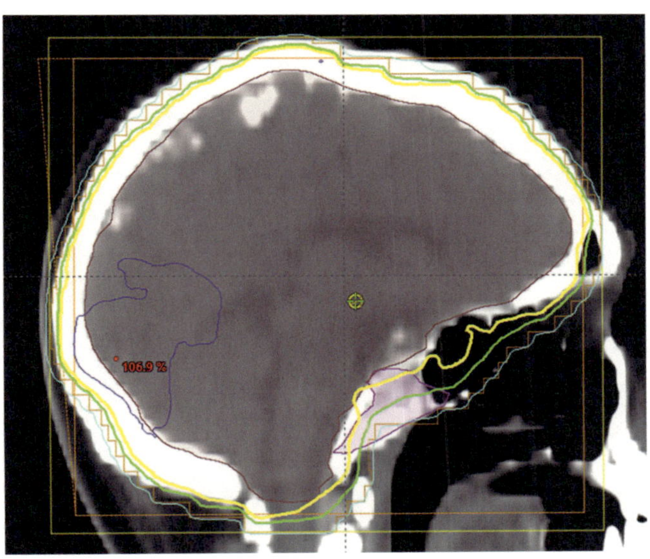

Figure 5.
Compromised coverage of the cranial nerves when the clivus is not fully contoured.

subsequently embedded into protocols, it takes time for the global radiation oncology community to adapt to changes in protocol. This was especially true in all disease areas as we transitioned to volumetric treatment planning using three-dimensional images to replace fluoroscopy. Over time, investigators have been successful in transitioning radiation therapy treatment planning processes into volumetric targeting, which is now exclusively embedded into the National Clinical Trials Network portfolio of clinical studies.

As technology of radiation therapy has progressively advanced, patients have benefitted from accompanying process improvements and favorable treatment outcomes. The incorporation of image guidance into modern radiation therapy care has afforded a greater degree of daily treatment reproducibility, generating confidence

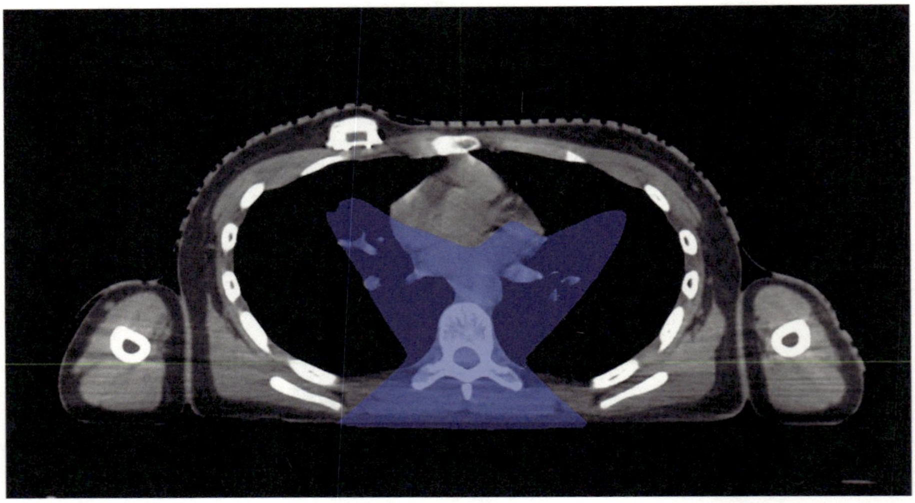

Figure 6.
Radiation dose to the spine with photon fields. Note the dose to central lung and cardiac structures.

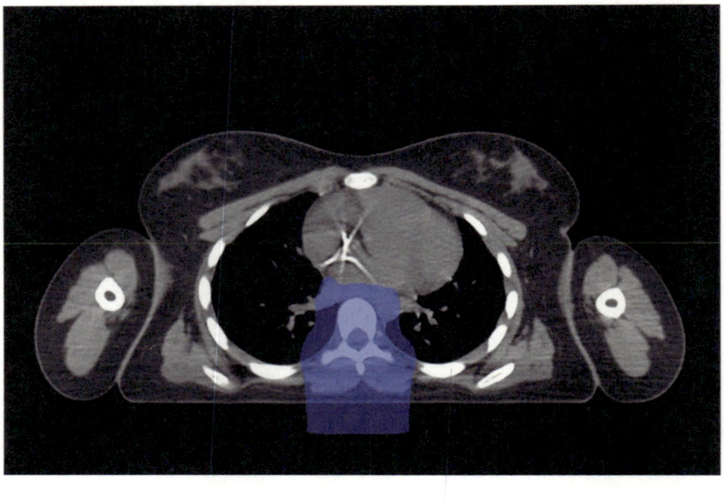

Figure 7.
Radiation fields to the spine with proton therapy. Note the decreased dose to lung and cardiac structures compared to the photon plan.

in decreasing expanded targets including the planning target volume of radiation therapy treatment fields, which decreases radiation dose to normal tissue. As proton therapy centers increase in number across the world, an increasing number of medulloblastoma patients are being treated with particle therapy. Protons do not have an exit dose, therefore, treating a spine field with protons eliminates unintended dose to cardiac, pulmonary, and additional normal tissue. Protons also permit decreased dose to growth segments of bony structures, allowing for less consequential impact on normal physiologic processes of growth and development. A comparison of dose to structures between protons and photons is presented in **Figures 6** and 7 [40–45].

7. Conclusions

Radiation therapy has played and continues to play an important role in the care of patients with medulloblastoma. Clinical trials have supported how best to optimize systemic therapy in this disease and will serve to determine how radiation dose and volume titration or augmentation can be performed to further enhance cure while decreasing normal tissue late treatment effects. Current technology permits selected areas of volume titration, and as functional imaging becomes incorporated into clinical trials, selected areas in the central nervous system can be contoured and treated with dose gradients further sparing normal tissue in vulnerable patients. Novel radiation delivery techniques including proton and particle therapies could also significantly improve the therapeutic ratio. The expansion of biomarker-driven therapies, coupled with the selected use of normal tissue-sparing radiation therapy techniques, offers considerable promise in further patient treatment stratification that stands to improve outcomes for patients with this disease therapeutic ratio [46–54].

Acknowledgements

This work was supported in part by the NCI Grant to the Imaging and Radiation Oncology Core, CA180803.

Conflict of interest

The authors declare no conflict of interest.

Author details

David Harris[1,2*], Jessica Yancey[1,2], Gavin Jones[1,2], Koren Smith[2], Sandy Kessel[2], Fran Laurie[2], Matthew Iandoli[2], Maryann Bishop-Jodoin[2], Yansong Geng[1], Linda Ding[1,2], Julie Trifone[1], Julia Hayden[2], Eric Ko[1,2] and Paul Rava[1,2]

1 UMass Memorial Health, Worcester, MA, United States

2 University of Massachusetts Chan Medical School, Worcester, MA, United States

*Address all correspondence to: david.harris@umassmemorial.org

References

[1] Packer RJ, Sutton LN, Elterman R, Lange B, Goldwein J, Nicholson HS, et al. Outcomeforchildrenwithmedulloblastoma treated with radiation and cisplatin, CCNU, and vincristine chemotherapy. Journal of Neurosurgery. 1994;**81**(5): 690-698. DOI: 10.3171/jns.1994.81.5.0690

[2] Bailey CC, Gnekow A, Wellek S, Jones M, Round C, Brown J, et al. Prospective randomised trial of chemotherapy given before radiotherapy in childhood medulloblastoma. International Society of Paediatric Oncology (SIOP) and the (German) Society of Paediatric Oncology (GPO): SIOP II. Medical and Pediatric Oncology. 1995;**25**(3):166-178. DOI: 10.1002/mpo.2950250303

[3] Packer RJ, Goldwein J, Nicholson HS, Vezina LG, Allen JC, Ris MD, et al. Treatment of children with medulloblastomas with reduced-dose craniospinal radiation therapy and adjuvant chemotherapy: A Children's cancer group study. Journal of Clinical Oncology. 1999;**17**(7):2127-2136. DOI: 10.1200/JCO.1999.17.7.2127

[4] Kortmann RD, Kühl J, Timmermann B, Mittler U, Urban C, Budach V, et al. Postoperative neoadjuvant chemotherapy before radiotherapy as compared to immediate radiotherapy followed by maintenance chemotherapy in the treatment of medulloblastoma in childhood: Results of the German prospective randomized trial HIT '91. International Journal of Radiation Oncology, Biology, Physics. 2000;**46**(2):269-279. DOI: 10.1016/S0360-3016(99)00369-7

[5] Taylor RE, Bailey CC, Robinson KJ, Weston CL, Ellison D, Ironside J, et al. Impact of radiotherapy parameters on outcome in the International Society of Paediatric Oncology/United Kingdom Children's Cancer Study Group PNET-3 study of preradiotherapy chemotherapy for M0-M1 medulloblastoma. International Journal of Radiation Oncology, Biology, Physics. 2004;**58**(4):1184-1193. DOI: 10.1016/j.ijrobp.2003.08.010

[6] Hoff KV, Hinkes B, Gerber NU, Deinlein F, Mittler U, Urban C, et al. Long-term outcome and clinical prognostic factors in children with medulloblastoma treated in the prospective randomised multicentre trial HIT'91. European Journal of Cancer. 2009;**45**(7):1209-1217. DOI: 10.1016/j.ejca.2009.01.015

[7] Cushing H. Experiences with the cerebellar medulloblastomas: Critical review. Acta Pathologica Microbiologica Scandinavica. 1930;**7**(1-2):1-86. DOI: 10.1111/j.1600-0463.1930.tb06503.x

[8] Paterson E, Farr RF. Cerebellar medulloblastoma: Treatment by irradiation of the whole central nervous system. Acta Radiologica. 1953;**39**(4):323-336. DOI: 10.1177/028418515303900407

[9] Smith CE, Long DM, Jones TK Jr, Levitt SH. Experiences in treating medulloblastoma at the University of Minnesota hospitals. Radiology. 1973;**109**(1):179-182. DOI: 10.1148/109.1.179

[10] Jenkin RD. Medulloblastoma in childhood: Radiation therapy. Canadian Medical Association Journal. 1969;**100**(2):51-53

[11] Bloom HJ, Wallace EN, Henk JM. The treatment and prognosis of

medulloblastoma in children. A study of 82 verified cases. The American Journal of Roentgenology, Radium Therapy, and Nuclear Medicine. 1969;**105**(1):43-62. DOI: 10.2214/ajr.105.1.43

[12] Chatty EM, Earle KM. Medulloblastoma. A report of 201 cases with emphasis on the relationship of histologic variants to survival. Cancer. 1971;**28**(4):977-983. DOI: 10.1002/1097-0142(1971)28:4<977::AID-CNCR2820280422>3.0.CO;2-7

[13] Ajithkumar T, Price S, Horan G, Burke A, Jefferies S. Prevention of radiotherapy-induced neurocognitive dysfunction in survivors of paediatric brain tumours: The potential role of modern imaging and radiotherapy techniques. The Lancet Oncology. 2017;**18**(2):e91-e100. DOI: 10.1016/S1470-2045(17)30030-X

[14] Al-Wassia RK, Ghassal NM, Naga A, Awad NA, Bahadur YA, Constantinescu C. Optimization of craniospinal irradiation for pediatric medulloblastoma using VMAT and IMRT. Journal of Pediatric Hematology/Oncology. 2015;**37**(7):e405-e411. DOI: 10.1097/MPH.0000000000000418

[15] Solit DB, Goldwein JW. Posterior fossa: Analysis of a popular technique for estimating the location in children with medulloblastoma. Radiology. 1995;**195**(3):697-698. DOI: 10.1148/radiology.195.3.7753996

[16] Noble DJ, Ajithkumar T, Lambert J, Gleeson I, Williams MV, Jefferies SJ. Highly conformal craniospinal radiotherapy techniques can underdose the cranial clinical target volume if leptomeningeal extension through skull base exit foramina is not contoured. Clinical Oncology (Royal College of Radiologists). 2017;**29**(7):439-447. DOI: 10.1016/j.clon.2017.02.013

[17] Ajithkumar T, Horan G, Padovani L, Thorp N, Timmermann B, Alapetite C, et al. SIOPE - brain tumor group consensus guideline on craniospinal target volume delineation for high-precision radiotherapy. Radiotherapy and Oncology. 2018;**128**(2):192-197. DOI: 10.1016/j.radonc.2018.04.016

[18] Seravalli E, Bosman M, Lassen-Ramshad Y, Vestergaard A, Oldenburger F, Visser J, et al. Dosimetric comparison of five different techniques for craniospinal irradiation across 15 European centers: Analysis on behalf of the SIOP-E-BTG (radiotherapy working group). Acta Oncologica. 2018;**57**(9):1240-1249. DOI: 10.1080/0284186X.2018.1465588

[19] Packer RJ, Zhou T, Holmes E, Vezina G, Gajjar A. Survival and secondary tumors in children with medulloblastoma receiving radiotherapy and adjuvant chemotherapy: Results of Children's Oncology Group trial A9961. Neuro-Oncology. 2013;**15**(1):97-103. DOI: 10.1093/neuonc/nos267

[20] Donahue B, Marymont MA, Kessel S, Iandoli MK, Fitzgerald T, Holmes E, et al. Radiation therapy quality in CCG/POG intergroup 9961: Implications for cranialspinal irradiation and the posterior fossa boost in future medulloblastoma trials. Frontiers in Oncology. 2012;**2**:185. DOI: 10.3389/fonc.2012.00185

[21] Michalski JM, Janss AJ, Vezina LG, Smith KS, Billups CA, Burger PC, et al. Children's oncology group phase III trial of reduced-dose and reduced-volume radiotherapy with chemotherapy for newly diagnosed average-risk medulloblastoma. Journal of Clinical Oncology. 2021;**39**(24):2685-2697. DOI: 10.1200/JCO.20.02730

[22] Carrie C, Grill J, Figarella-Branger D, Bernier V, Padovani L, Habrand JL, et al.

Online quality control, hyperfractionated radiotherapy alone and reduced boost volume for standard risk medulloblastoma: Long-term results of MSFOP 98. Journal of Clinical Oncology. 2009;**27**(11):1879-1883. DOI: 10.1200/JCO.2008.18.6437

[23] Dietzsch S, Braesigk A, Seidel C, Remmele J, Kitzing R, Schlender T, et al. Pretreatment central quality control for craniospinal irradiation in non-metastatic medulloblastoma: First experiences of the German radiotherapy quality control panel in the SIOP PNET5 MB trial. Strahlentherapie und Onkologie. 2021;**197**(8):674-682. DOI: 10.1007/s00066-020-01707-8

[24] Dietzsch S, Braesigk A, Seidel C, Remmele J, Kitzing R, Schlender T, et al. Types of deviation and review criteria in pretreatment central quality control of tumor bed boost in medulloblastoma-an analysis of the German Radiotherapy Quality Control Panel in the SIOP PNET5 MB trial. Strahlentherapie und Onkologie. 2021;**198**(3):282-290. DOI: 10.1007/s00066-021-01822-0

[25] Bouffet E. Management of high-risk medulloblastoma. Neuro-Chirurgie. 2021;**67**(1):61-68. DOI: 10.1016/j.neuchi.2019.05.007

[26] Dangouloff-Ros V, Varlet P, Levy R, Beccaria K, Puget S, Dufour C, et al. Imaging features of medulloblastoma: Conventional imaging, diffusion-weighted imaging, perfusion-weighted imaging, and spectroscopy: From general features to subtypes and characteristics. Neuro-Chirurgie. 2021;**67**(1):6-13. DOI: 10.1016/j.neuchi.2017.10.003

[27] Dasgupta A, Maitre M, Pungavkar S, Gupta T. Magnetic resonance imaging in the contemporary management of medulloblastoma: Current and emerging applications. Methods in Molecular Biology. 2022;**2423**:187-214. DOI: 10.1007/978-1-0716-1952-0

[28] Phi JH, Lee J, Wang KC, Cho BK, Kim IO, Park CK, et al. Cerebrospinal fluid M staging for medulloblastoma: Reappraisal of Chang's M staging based on the CSF flow. Neuro-Oncology. 2011;**13**(3):334-344. DOI: 10.1093/neuonc/noq171

[29] Louis DN, Perry A, Reifenberger G, von Deimling A, Figarella-Branger D, Cavenee WK, et al. The 2016 world health organization classification of tumors of the central nervous system: A summary. Acta Neuropathologica. 2016;**131**(6):803-820. DOI: 10.1007/s00401-016-1545-1

[30] Chang CH, Housepian EM, Herbert C Jr. An operative staging system and a megavoltage radiotherapeutic technic for cerebellar medulloblastomas. Radiology. 1969;**93**(6):1351-1359. DOI: 10.1148/93.6.1351

[31] Taylor MD, Northcott PA, Korshunov A, Remke M, Cho YJ, Clifford SC, et al. Molecular subgroups of medulloblastoma: The current consensus. Acta Neuropathologica. 2012;**123**(4):465-472. DOI: 10.1007/s00401-011-0922-z

[32] Ramaswamy V, Remke M, Bouffet E, Bailey S, Clifford SC, Doz F, et al. Risk stratification of childhood medulloblastoma in the molecular era: The current consensus. Acta Neuropathologica. 2016;**131**(6):821-831. DOI: 10.1007/s00401-016-1569-6

[33] Reddy N, Ellison DW, Soares BP, Carson KA, Huisman TAGM, Patay Z. Pediatric posterior fossa medulloblastoma: The role of diffusion imaging in identifying molecular groups. Journal of Neuroimaging. 2020;**30**(4):503-511. DOI: 10.1111/jon.12704

[34] Zhang M, Wong SW, Wright JN, Wagner MW, Toescu S, Han M, et al. MRI radiogenomics of pediatric medulloblastoma: A multicenter study. Radiology. 2022;**304**(2):406-416. DOI: 10.1148/radiol.212137

[35] Carrie C, Hoffstetter S, Gomez F, Moncho V, Doz F, Alapetite C, et al. Impact of targeting deviations on outcome in medulloblastoma: Study of the French Society of Pediatric Oncology (SFOP). International Journal of Radiation Oncology, Biology, Physics. 1999;**45**(2):435-439. DOI: 10.1016/S0360-3016(99)00200-X

[36] Kortmann RD, Timmermann B, Kühl J, Willich N, Flentje M, Meisner C, et al. HIT'91 (prospective, co-operative study for the treatment of malignant brain tumors in childhood): Accuracy and acute toxicity of the irradiation of the craniospinal axis. Results of the quality assurance program. Strahlentherapie und Onkologie. 1999;**175**(4):162-169. DOI: 10.1007/BF02742358

[37] Chojnacka M, Skowrońska-Gardas A. Medulloblastoma in childhood: Impact of radiation technique upon the outcome of treatment. Pediatric Blood & Cancer. 2004;**42**(2):155-160. DOI: 10.1002/pbc.10401

[38] Jereb B, Reid A, Ahuja RK. Patterns of failure in patients with medulloblastoma. Cancer. 1982;**50**(12):2941-2947. DOI: 10.1002/1097-0142(19821215)50:12<2941::aid-cncr2820501239>3.0.co;2-6

[39] Miralbell R, Bleher A, Huguenin P, Ries G, Kann R, Mirimanoff RO, et al. Pediatric medulloblastoma: Radiation treatment technique and patterns of failure. International Journal of Radiation Oncology, Biology, Physics. 1997;**37**(3):523-529. DOI: 10.1016/s0360-3016(96)00569-x

[40] Yock TI, Yeap BY, Ebb DH, Weyman E, Eaton BR, Sherry NA, et al. Long-term toxic effects of proton radiotherapy for paediatric medulloblastoma: A phase 2 single-arm study. The Lancet Oncology. 2016;**17**(3):287-298. DOI: 10.1016/S1470-2045(15)00167-9

[41] Eaton BR, Esiashvili N, Kim S, Weyman EA, Thornton LT, Mazewski C, et al. Clinical outcomes among children with standard-risk medulloblastoma treated with proton and photon radiation therapy: A comparison of disease control and overall survival. International Journal of Radiation Oncology, Biology, Physics. 2016;**94**(1):133-138. DOI: 10.1016/j.ijrobp.2015.09.014

[42] Paulino AC, Mahajan A, Ye R, Grosshans DR, Fatih Okcu M, Su J, et al. Ototoxicity and cochlear sparing in children with medulloblastoma: Proton vs. photon radiotherapy. Radiotherapy and Oncology. 2018;**128**(1):128-132. DOI: 10.1016/j.radonc.2018.01.002

[43] Bernier V, Klein O. Late effects of craniospinal irradiation for medulloblastomas in paediatric patients. Neuro-Chirurgie. 2021;**67**(1):83-86. DOI: 10.1016/j.neuchi.2018.01.006

[44] Ning MS, Perkins SM, Dewees T, Shinohara ET. Evidence of high mortality in long term survivors of childhood medulloblastoma. Journal of Neuro-Oncology. 2015;**122**(2):321-327. DOI: 10.1007/s11060-014-1712-y

[45] Bavle A, Tewari S, Sisson A, Chintagumpala M, Anderson M, Paulino AC. Meta-analysis of the incidence and patterns of second neoplasms after photon craniospinal irradiation in children with medulloblastoma. Pediatric Blood & Cancer. 2018;**65**(8):e27095. DOI: 10.1002/pbc.27095

[46] Archer TC, Ehrenberger T, Mundt F, Gold MP, Krug K, Mah CK, et al. Proteomics, post-translational modifications, and integrative analyses reveal molecular heterogeneity within medulloblastoma subgroups. Cancer Cell. 2018;**34**(3):396-410.e8. DOI: 10.1016/j.ccell.2018.08.004

[47] Archer TC, Mahoney EL, Pomeroy SL. Medulloblastoma: Molecular classification-based personal therapeutics. Neurotherapeutics. 2017;**14**(2):265-273. DOI: 10.1007/s13311-017-0526-y

[48] Northcott PA, Buchhalter I, Morrissy AS, Hovestadt V, Weischenfeldt J, Ehrenberger T, et al. The whole-genome landscape of medulloblastoma subtypes. Nature. 2017;**547**(7663):311-317. DOI: 10.1038/nature22973

[49] Hein AL, Ouellette MM, Yan Y. Radiation-induced signaling pathways that promote cancer cell survival (review). International Journal of Oncology. 2014;**45**(5):1813-1819. DOI: 10.3892/ijo.2014.2614

[50] de Bont JM, Packer RJ, Michiels EM, den Boer ML, Pieters R. Biological background of pediatric medulloblastoma and ependymoma: A review from a translational research perspective. Neuro-Oncology. 2008;**10**(6):1040-1060. DOI: 10.1215/15228517-2008-059

[51] Nakamura M, Masutomi K, Kyo S, Hashimoto M, Maida Y, Kanaya T, et al. Efficient inhibition of human telomerase reverse transcriptase expression by RNA interference sensitizes cancer cells to ionizing radiation and chemotherapy. Human Gene Therapy. 2005;**16**(7):859-868. DOI: 10.1089/hum.2005.16.859

[52] Patties I, Kortmann RD, Menzel F, Glasow A. Enhanced inhibition of clonogenic survival of human medulloblastoma cells by multimodal treatment with ionizing irradiation, epigenetic modifiers, and differentiation-inducing drugs. Journal of Experimental & Clinical Cancer Research. 2016;**35**(1):94. DOI: 10.1186/s13046-016-0376-1

[53] Chang Q, Pang JC, Li J, Hu L, Kong X, Ng HK. Molecular analysis of PinX1 in medulloblastomas. International Journal of Cancer. 2004;**109**(2):309-314. DOI: 10.1002/ijc.11689

[54] Schiff JP, Lee Y, Wang Y, Perkins SM, Kessel SK, Fitzgerald TJ, et al. An analysis of major target deviations in craniospinal irradiation treatment plans for patients with intermediate risk medulloblastoma within a phase 3 clinical trial (Children's Oncology Group Study ACNS0331). Advances in Radiation Oncology. 2022;**8**(1):101083. DOI: 10.1016/j.adro.2022.101083

Chapter 6

Imaging and Medulloblastoma

Hebah Abudawaba, Vinaya Rajahraman, Maryann Bishop-Jodoin and John M. Buatti

Abstract

As therapy for medulloblastoma has matured, imaging has evolved and is now an essential component of the care of patients with medulloblastoma. Imaging defines the extent of disease at presentation and is the primary vehicle for staging patients to ensure the correct therapy is applied to the patient. Radiation therapy has moved away from anatomical definitions of targets to image-guided target volumes; therefore, imaging platforms are essential for both targeting disease and accurate daily positioning for therapy. Imaging is now our primary vehicle post-treatment to determine both tumor control and quantification of toxicity. In this chapter, we review the modern role of imaging in this disease and in clinical trials.

Keywords: medulloblastoma, imaging, magnetic resonance, clinical trials, imaging/radiation therapy

1. Introduction

Central nervous system (CNS) tumors (tumors of the brain and spine) are a serious health problem among different age groups. They constitute the most common solid malignancies in children and adolescents (ages 0–19 years), with an average annual incidence rate of malignant and non-malignant brain and other CNS tumors of 6.2 per 100,000 population [1]. In addition, approximately 28.3% of all brain and other CNS tumors are malignant, and 71.7% are non-malignant [1]. Medulloblastoma (MB) is the most common malignant brain tumor in children and adolescents, accounting for 20% of all pediatric brain tumors [2]. For those 18 years and older, MB accounts for 1–3% of primary CNS tumors and about 15–20% of all MB patients [3, 4]. Originating mostly from the cerebellum in the posterior fossa, MB is a primitive embryonal tumor and histologically classified as a World Health Organization (WHO) grade IV tumor [5, 6].

In oncology, imaging plays a critical role in the diagnosis (analysis of the lesion), staging (determining the amount of disease), quantifying residual tumor after surgery (extent of resection), delineating the radiotherapy (RT) target volumes and organs-at-risk (OAR), assessing post-treatment response, and follow-up surveillance and monitoring. Magnetic resonance imaging (MRI), a noninvasive imaging technique, does not use radiation but relies on a magnetic field and computer-generated radio waves. With its ability to provide detailed multiparametric images of the structures and organs in the body, including the entire craniospinal axis, MRI is the recommended first-line imaging modality for suspected brain tumors, including MB [7].

Advances in neuroimaging have improved the accuracy of diagnosing CNS tumors; for example, computed tomography (CT) may be helpful in delineating calcification typically seen in craniopharyngioma and malignant germ cell tumors (GCTs). Perfusion, diffusion, and diffusion tensor MR imaging add to diagnostic capabilities. In suprasellar and pineal region lesions, positron emission tomography (PET), single photon emission tomography (SPECT), magnetic resonance spectroscopy (MRS), and magnetoencephalography are used to evaluate the type and grade of tumor as well as differentiating tumor progression from radiation-related changes (e.g., intralesional necrosis) [8].

It is commonly accepted that imaging suggests underlying disease biology, showing complex biological processes such as gene expression, proliferation, metabolism, and angiogenesis, and is utilized as classifiers and prognostic biomarkers in the emerging radiomics/radiogenomics field [7].

2. History of medical imaging

Wilhelm Conrad Roentgen discovered X-rays in November of 1895 and thus began the field of medical imaging [9–11]. Skull radiographs offered limited capacity to define soft-tissue changes, and their utility was primarily in detecting tumors with calcification, bone destruction, or abnormalities visible only at advanced stages of disease [4–6]. Nonetheless, this newfound ability to visualize internal structures without invasive procedures was invaluable and led to many advancements in the neuro-oncology field of patient care.

Pneumoencephalography and ventriculography were the next advancements and were developed after Walter E. Dandy observed free intraperitoneal air-outlined abdominal organs and applied a similar concept to the brain in 1918–1919 [10–12]. These modalities marked the advent of contrast studies for the CNS and enabled the diagnosis of more intracranial pathologies compared to X-rays alone [12, 13].

Though Egas Moniz was unable to opacify the brain directly with a radiopaque contrast agent, he did succeed in visualizing the cerebral arteries using sodium iodide and created cerebral angiography in 1927 [10, 12, 14, 15]. As cerebral angiography was continuously refined by experts over the next few decades, it became a valuable tool for precisely locating cerebral masses based on vascular shifts and enabled the development of differential diagnoses of tumors based on angiographic patterns of the masses [10, 12, 16, 17].

Established in 1961, PET could detect positron-emitting radionuclides and display three-dimensional (3D) images [2]. Initially, 2-deoxy-2-[18F]fluoro-D-glucose (18F-FDG) was used as a radiotracer to demonstrate the higher metabolic activity of tumor cells compared to normal brain tissue; however, the high background uptake of 18F-FDG in normal brain limited its practical utility for CNS tumors. The more recent advent of amino acid PET tracers was found to have greater sensitivity and normal tissue contrast given their lower uptake in normal gray matter compared to 18F-FDG [18, 19]. These tracers also served to identify areas of DNA synthesis in tumor populations, which is often underappreciated with current imaging modalities.

The introduction of computed tomography (CT) by Sir Godfrey Hounsfield, a computer engineer, in 1971 marked the beginning of a new era in neuroimaging, allowing for the direct, noninvasive visualization of the brain's internal soft-tissue structure [12, 20, 21]. In the United States, the first CT scanners were introduced in 1973 at the Mayo Clinic and Massachusetts General Hospital (MGH) [22, 23]. Iodinated contrast material also aided in visualizing abnormalities in the vasculature and the meninges [12, 23, 24]. Compared to older modalities, CT scans led to a reduction of cost, time, and risk to the patient compared to more invasive methods like angiography [25]. With the introduction of CT, the use of pneumoencephalography, ventriculography, and angiography decreased exponentially for the diagnosis of brain tumors [12, 26].

CT scans were not the only type of imaging to revolutionize neuroradiology. Around the same time that CT scans were progressing, Raymond Damadian demonstrated that nuclear magnetic resonance (NMR) could help distinguish healthy tissue from tumors in 1971 [12, 27]. In 1973, Paul Lauterbur was able to use MRI to capture images of a mouse [12, 28]. A few years later, Peter Mansfield was able to develop mathematical algorithms enabling rapid imaging with MR, leading to the first human MR images of a finger and chest being reported in 1977 [10].

Despite the poor spatial resolution of the earliest brain MR images, their contrast resolution surpassed that of CT scans [12, 29]. MRI allowed for scanning multiple planes and the use of various pulse sequences to highlight different tissue contrasts [12, 30]. The introduction of gadolinium-based contrast agents in the 1980s enhanced MR's capacity to identify small lesions, like pituitary microadenomas and small vestibular schwannomas, which were not previously visible on CT or non-contrast MR images [12, 31–33]. Though CT scans are still largely used in emergent settings, as MRI technology has evolved, it has become the primary choice for brain imaging in most situations, as it can provide clearer visualizations of both normal and abnormal structures and often facilitates precise histological diagnoses [12, 29, 34].

3. Current MRI methods for brain tumors

Conventional anatomic MRI remains the primary imaging technique used in neuro-oncology [34–36]. MRI plays a crucial role in the initial evaluation of brain tumors by identifying the location of lesions, parenchymal tissue involvement, and the mass effect of lesions within and abutting the brain, vasculature, and ventricles [36, 37]. Though it can be difficult to determine the exact histological type of tumor based on imaging alone, MRI can narrow the possibilities when combined with factors such as tumor location, history of prior radiation, symptom duration, patient age, and presence of existing malignancy [36].

The current consensus standardized MRI protocol for brain tumors includes the following sequences, all conducted on a minimum of a 1.5 tesla (T) MR system, with more advanced 3 T systems commonly used today: 3D pre-contrast T1-weighted imaging, axial two-dimensional (2D) fluid-attenuated inversion recovery (FLAIR), axial 2D diffusion-weighted imaging (DWI), axial 2D gadolinium contrast-enhanced T2-weighted imaging, and 3D gadolinium contrast-enhanced T1-weighted imaging [36, 38]. In the case of challenges such as technical limitations or time constraints, 2-D sequences may be used in lieu of 3-D sequences [36]. In addition, the utilization of perfusion imaging and spectroscopic imaging has also increased in frequency, although these methods require specialized expertise and processing methods to implement effectively. Such methods continue to evolve and offer the potential to further narrow the differential diagnosis and to effectively evaluate physiologic changes that may impact prognosis and response.

Pre- and post-contrast MR imaging has been the standard for detecting, anatomically defining, and assessing the response of malignant brain tumors [36, 39]. Multiple studies have associated neovascularization and structural abnormalities of the vasculature with leakage of the gadolinium contrast agent into the affected tumor tissue, which can shorten the T1 relaxation time, from the vascular to extravascular space, enhancing the areas around active tumor sites on imaging [36, 38]. This is sometimes associated with more aggressive malignancies, although this is not universally true. The T2/FLAIR hyperintense signal often surrounds an enhancing tumor core, also known as peritumoral edema. This can be purely vasogenic edema (reactive fluid accumulation without tumor cells, often seen around metastases or non-infiltrative extra-axial tumors like meningiomas) or infiltrative edema (a mix of vasogenic edema and infiltrating tumor cells) [36, 40, 41]. The differences in these edema patterns may be difficult to distinguish. The DWI MR sequence can evaluate a multitude of tumor characteristics, including tissue cellularity, hypoxic tumor regions, peritumoral edema, the condition of white matter tracts, and postoperative injury by exploring the random (Brownian) movement of water molecules within the brain [42, 43]. Lower apparent diffusion coefficient (ADC) values are calculated from DWI and reflect decreased water diffusivity, suggesting tumors with high cellularity, such as MB or lymphoma [44, 45].

Advanced imaging modalities beyond the standard anatomic MRI sequences can also be helpful for the diagnosis of brain tumors. MR perfusion techniques can be used, such as T2-based dynamic susceptibility contrast (DSC) and T1-based dynamic-contrast enhanced (DCE) perfusion-weighted imaging (PWI) [36]. DSC imaging, more commonly used than DCE perfusion, relies on identifying signal loss caused by susceptibility following the administration of intravenous gadolinium contrast. Using a signal intensity time curve, relative cerebral blood volume (rCBV) and other perfusion parameters are calculated; elevated rCBV is indicative of tumors and is a marker of angiogenesis [36, 46]. MRS analyzes the chemical composition of a tissue volume and displays it as an NMR spectrum [47]. With the presence of brain tumors, MR spectra would show a decrease in normal neuronal metabolites (N-acetyl aspartate—NAA) and increased cellular turnover (Cho-choline) [48]. Diffusion tensor imaging (DTI) uses the tissue diffusivity and fiber direction in order to outline the 3D shape of fiber tracts based on diffusion in and around tumors and is helpful in presurgical planning for tumor resection [36, 49]. Decreased blood oxygen level dependent (BOLD) imaging utilizes the ratio of deoxyhemoglobin to oxyhemoglobin in order to define functional MRI (fMRI) areas that can be seen in the brain cortex when certain tasks are performed and can also help in presurgical planning to demonstrate how areas around tumors are active or eloquent for specific neurologic activities [36, 50]. Additionally, 3D T2-weighted and 3D post-contrast T1-weighted spoiled gradient echo sequences are essential for neuro-navigation and planning presurgical biopsies since they offer high-resolution, 3D volumetric images that are most useful in directing interventions [36]. All sequences play a role in defining target volumes of interest, as each provides a different window into tissues at risk for disease, and each can be applied to demonstrate a response to therapy or disease progression.

4. Current status of radiomics

Radiomics is a relatively new quantitative method for analyzing medical imaging, designed to enhance the utility of information available to clinicians by applying advanced mathematical techniques and artificial intelligence (AI) to imaging data [51]. Radiomics is based on the concept that visual inspection of images is not sufficient to gather all the potential information within the imaging data to define disease-specific processes; thus, with mathematical analysis, more detailed textural information can be both quantified and made objective [51–53]. Additionally, radiomics can combine data from multiple imaging modalities, such as CT scans, multiple sequences on MRI, and PET scans, as opposed to considering each modality on its own [51].

An important first step in radiomics analysis is accurate image segmentation of the tumor and normal tissue of interest which involves either defining the region of interest (ROI) in 2D or the volume of interest (VOI) in 3D, as these are where radiomic features are calculated [51, 54]. Traditionally, this was done manually and resulted in significant variability between investigators. More recently, automated, and specifically AI-driven, methods have improved both the efficiency and consistency of this process. Step two is image processing, in which images are ideally made optimally homogeneous regarding characteristics such as pixel spacing, bins of the gray-level histogram, gray-level intensities, and more [51]. This harmonization process is problematic in using data from multiple institutions or from different machines (and potentially vendors) within a single institution. Making image acquisition more consistent and establishing rigorous quality assurance methods in imaging will help mitigate issues related to inherent differences in the images. Step three is radiomic feature extraction, where the gray levels or imaging characteristics within the ROI and VOI are quantified using mathematically defined descriptors/features such as intensity, shape, texture, and radial features [51, 55]. Step four, called dimension reduction or feature selection, attempts to reduce the number of features used by selecting those that are most predictive of the desired outcome and excluding those that are least informative or potentially overlapping with the most significant features. Once a reduction is achieved, step five builds the machine learning and statistical models. Having too many features may lead to an increase in the false discovery rate, and overlapping features may lead to overfitting in the models that are developed [55]. The interaction of statisticians with AI and deep learning experts is essential in developing informative radiomic analyses from imaging data. Similar processes are in development for the application of radiation therapy treatment plans as well as scoring the strength or compliance of the plan to clinical trial guidelines.

Radiomics for the evaluation of brain tumors is most commonly applied to MR imaging data and often with multi-parameter/multi-sequence data [56]. Radiomic techniques can help determine histopathologic classification and grading of tumors as well as distinguish different types of tumors, such as metastases from primary brain tumors [56, 57]. Studies have reported using radiomic analysis to estimate tumor proliferation indices, like Ki67, and for separating vasogenic edema from infiltrative edema [56, 58, 59]. Multiple studies have reported the potential to utilize radiomics to predict molecular phenotypes of tumors, such as p53 or isocitrate dehydrogenase 1 mutation status in gliomas [56, 60, 61]. Radiation necrosis and pseudoprogression may be distinguishable from tumor progression, recurrence, or metastases using radiomic analysis [56, 62]. Radiomics may also be used to predict the response of brain metastases to stereotactic radiosurgery [56]. This is essential moving forward, as often tissue necrosis and disease progression are difficult to define and identify from images post therapy.

5. Current state of the art for diagnosis and staging of medulloblastoma

MB is the most common pediatric malignant CNS tumor and is now classified into four molecular subgroups: group 1 - wingless activated (WNT), group 2 - sonic hedgehog (SHH), group 3, and group 4. Each subgroup is associated with a distinct origin of development, transcriptional profile, and clinical behavior.

In many parts of the world, CT may be used as the index imaging for suspected MB. On non-enhanced CT, the tumor appears hyperdense compared with the surrounding unaffected normal cerebellum [63–65]. Other features commonly associated are peritumoral edema represented as a hypodense region and hydrocephalus with dilation of the third and lateral ventricles. Enhancement can be variable on contrast-enhanced CT, although the majority will show some degree of uptake. Other associated features that can be seen on CT are calcification, cystic spaces, or rarely hemorrhages. For a suggestive CT scan, a preoperative contrast-enhanced MRI of the brain and spine is recommended in suspected MB [66].

On non-contrast T1-weighted images, MB is generally isointense, although some additional features may be appreciated, such as focal areas of hyperintensity (hemorrhage, calcifications) or hypointensity (necrosis, cyst) within the tumor.

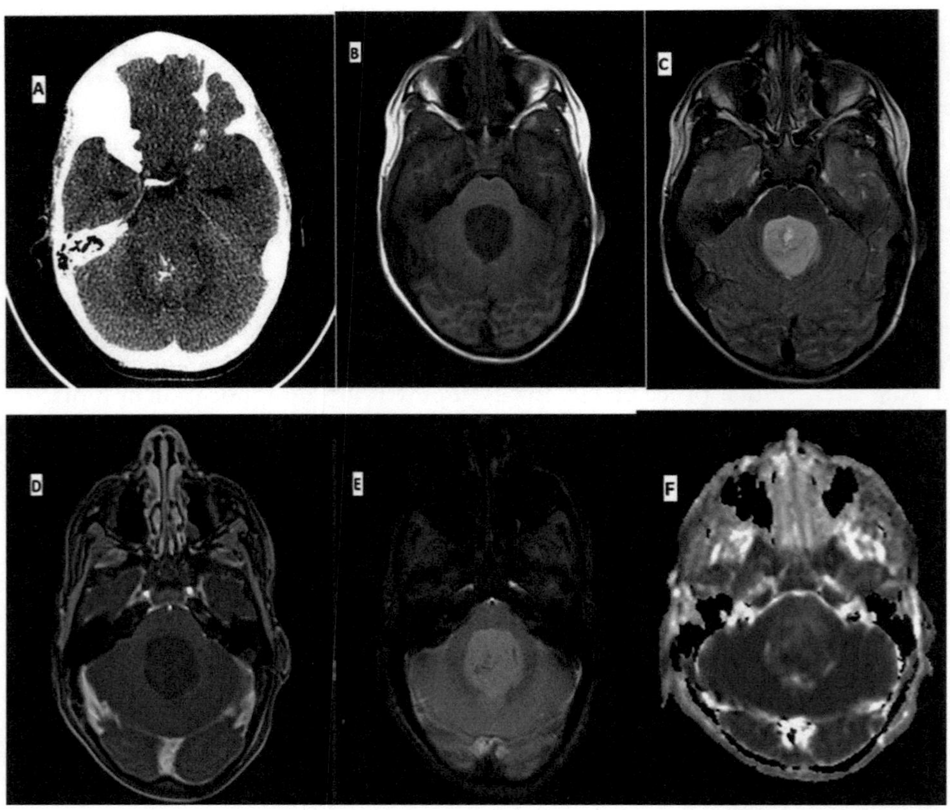

Figure 1.
Example of non-SHH/non-WNT MB in a 7-year-old boy. A large, slightly hyperdense cerebellar mass with centric hyperdensities (calcification versus hemorrhage) (A). The lesion appears hypointense on T1W with centric cystic hypointensities (B) and hyperintense on T2W with central cystic hyperintensities (C). On T1C the mass was non-enhancing (D) and did demonstrate restricted diffusion (E and F).

On T2-weighted images, the densely packed cellular component of the tumor is significantly hyperintense compared to the normal cerebellum. On the T2W MRI, it is important that the tumor characteristics are defined based on the solid portion of the tumor features, excluding the surrounding bright hyperintense regions representing edema. Necrosis and cysts are seen as bright signals. Calcification and hemorrhage appear as areas with hypointense signals. With these features, MB appears heterogeneous on T2 sequences [7]. Nonetheless, MB displays restricted diffusion on diffusion-weighted imaging. Following intravenous gadolinium, MB shows significant but variable and heterogeneous contrast enhancement. On post-contrast T1W images, MB with extensive nodularity (MBEN) can be identified as homogeneously enhancing grape-like nodular structures [67]. With the propensity of neuroaxis spread in MB, sagittal fat-suppressed T1 post-contrast MRI of the spine is recommended to rule out leptomeningeal metastasis for accurate staging (**Figure 1**).

At initial presentation, 20–40% of patients with MB have metastatic disease on neuroaxis staging [63, 67, 68]. The range of metastases includes cerebrospinal fluid (CSF), posterior fossa, supratentorial brain, spinal drop metastases, or diffuse leptomeningeal disease. Even though MB is the most common primary CNS tumor associated with extra neuroaxis metastasis (ENM), the reported incidence (2–5%) is rare, with <1% having ENM at presentation [68, 69]. Response Assessment in Pediatric Neuro-Oncology (RAPNO) guidelines recommend a screening MR of the spine immediately after brain MRI, without additional contrast, as the recommended sequences (T1W and T2W) can be acquired within 45 minutes of the initial gadolinium injection [70]. Typical sites of intracranial metastases include the infundibulum, suprachiasmatic recess, subependymal region of the lateral ventricles, basal cisterns, ventricular recess, and vermis [63]. Disease in the spine may manifest as nerve root thickening, thecal sac irregularity, cord enlargement, and nodular or laminar deposits.

Disease phase	Descriptive role of MRI
Diagnosis and staging	• Recommended first-line imaging modality for suspected brain tumors, including MB. • Recommended preoperative sagittal fat-suppressed post-contrast screening spinal MRI for neuroaxis staging. • MRI features (location, intensity, contrast enhancement, perifocal edema, cyst, necrosis, calcification, hemorrhage, diffusion characteristics, and leptomeningeal metastases) can reliably differentiate MB from other posterior fossa masses. • Pre-operatively identify molecular subgroups with implications on neurosurgical decisions. • Intraoperative MRI may maximize resection and minimize residual tumor.
Extent of resection	• Postoperative MRI confirms the extent of resection and accurately quantifies residual tumor. • Residual tumor > = 1.5 cm^2 is traditionally categorized as a high-risk disease. • Recommended postoperative MRI within 24–48 hours of surgery. If not, 2–3 weeks after surgery to allow postoperative changes and ischemia to resolve, which could interfere with correctly interpreting the MRI. • Recommend postoperative screening for accurate spinal staging if a preoperative MRI of the spine is not performed.
RT planning	• Accurate tumor bed mapping and localization during RT planning for tumor bed boost. • Accurate delineation of OAR during RT planning (for craniospinal RT and tumor bed boost).

Disease phase	Descriptive role of MRI
Response assessment	• Recommend neuroaxis MRI 4 weeks after adjuvant therapy for response assessment (initially after completing RT with or without concurrent chemotherapy) and subsequently after completing adjuvant systemic chemotherapy. • In infant MB (treated with systemic chemotherapy to defer RT) and patients on pre-RT chemotherapy for widely metastatic MB, MRI is recommended periodically on treatment (every 2–3 cycles) to assess disease status and detect progression/recurrence early, if any.
Surveillance and monitoring	• After completing therapy, surveillance MRI is recommended periodically (3–6 months through 5 years and annually for 10 years) to detect progression/recurrence. • Recommended MRI to be done promptly in patients with any new-onset neurologic symptoms and/or clinical/neurological worsening. Follow-up spinal MRI is recommended, particularly in patients with high-risk/metastatic disease, large-cell/anaplastic histology, and subgroups 3 or 4. If intracranial disease is suspected clinically, an MRI of the brain and spine should be done. • Surveillance MRI assists in detecting and monitoring long-term complications such as diffuse white matter changes, vasculopathy including cavernomas, cerebral atrophy, and second malignant neoplasm.
Radiomics and radiogenomics	• Recent studies utilizing multiparametric MRI have shown the potential for preoperative identification of molecular MB subgroups based on radiomic and/or semantic features. Prediction accuracy for SHH and Group 4 tumors is quite high but currently suboptimal and unacceptably low for WNT and Group 3 MB. • Future predictive studies generating imaging signatures (including advanced MRI techniques, functional MRI, and machine learning approaches).

Table 1.
The roles and applications of MRI in managing MB.

For patients with a negative MRI of the spine, microscopic disease must be ruled out with CSF malignant cell cytology. In a study [71] involving children with MB and other primitive neuroectodermal tumors, using spinal MRI and CSF cytology revealed leptomeningeal disease in 14–18% of patients that would have otherwise been missed if only one evaluation had been done. This will influence the treatment plan and alter the dose the individual would have received for the fluid pathways and spine in the study.

The applications and roles of MRI for diagnosis, staging, quantifying residual disease, post-treatment response assessment, periodic surveillance, and prediction of the molecular subgrouping in managing MB are summarized in **Table 1** [67].

6. Differential diagnosis of medulloblastoma and molecular subgroups

MB arises in the posterior fossa; however, posterior fossa tumors in the pediatric population include MB, ependymoma, pilocytic astrocytoma, brainstem glioma, and uncommon varieties of brain tumors, “non-MB primitive embryonal tumors,” such as atypical teratoid/rhabdoid tumor (AT/RT) and embryonal tumor with multilayered rosettes (ETMR). AT/RT, a variant of malignant embryonal tumor (WHO grade IV), has an aggressive biology and, on imaging, forms a similar appearance to MB. However, AT/RT most commonly affects infants (typically <3 years of age) [72, 73]. Usual presentation is a heterogeneously enhancing mass in the midline posterior fossa with necrosis and is often associated with hemorrhage, differentiating it from MB [7]. With the evolution of radiomics, additional morphological and textural features can be incorporated to differentiate between the two, which will be explained later on in this chapter.

Each post-fossa tumor is managed with a different approach; for example, ependymoma is a very "surgical" tumor, as its prognosis is most heavily dependent on the completeness of the resection. Pilocytic astrocytoma is also ideally completely resected, but in certain circumstances may intentionally be treated with more limited resection due to its location and anticipated relatively benign course. Maximum safe surgical resection is also the standard of treatment in medulloblastoma, and adjuvant therapies, including chemotherapy and RT, will be largely determined based on the ultimate risk stratification defined by the residual tumor and pathological subtype. Despite these tumors showing overlapping characteristics on conventional MRI scans, imaging features such as anatomic tumor location, tumor morphology, ADC, or spectroscopy are considered helpful during the diagnostic radiological process to differentiate between these tumors and can influence the preplanning decision regarding the extent of the surgical resection needed.

Ependymomas are the most common posterior fossa tumors associated with calcification, with punctate calcifications seen in nearly 50% of patients [7]. An additional tool to distinguish between MB and ependymomas is identifying the epicenter of the tumor. The epicenter of the tumor should be used to classify it as "midline" (vermis/brainstem) or "lateralized" (cerebellar hemisphere). Approximately 25–30% of MBs have hemispheric locations (more common in adults) and are generally associated with desmoplastic histology and the SHH subgroup [67, 74–78]. Characterizing the tumor epicenter on the horizontal and vertical axes can help in distinguishing it from other posterior fossa tumors. For categorizing the horizontal location, axial and coronal images are helpful, and both T1W and T2W sequences should be studied. For categorizing tumor location on the vertical axis, sagittal and coronal scans are helpful. The tumor epicenter is categorized in relation to the center of the fourth ventricle and classified as superior, central, or inferior (**Figure 2**). Tumors located superiorly are seen more frequently in MB, while tumors located inferiorly are seen more frequently in ependymoma. Though MB arising inferior to the center of the fourth ventricle is less frequently observed in clinical practice, it is specific for group 4 MB [7].

The classic appearance of a cerebellar pilocytic astrocytoma includes a large cyst in the cerebellum with a mural nodule [65, 79, 80]. Usually, the mural nodule shows bright homogenous contrast uptake, although the cyst wall may be associated with a variable degree of enhancement (**Figure 3**).

Brainstem gliomas constitute a variety of astrocytic tumors, including diffuse intrinsic pontine glioma, dorsal exophytic tumors, cervicomedullary junction astrocytoma, and focal tectal plate gliomas. Diffusion tensor imaging (DTI) is an MRI-based technique that assesses water diffusion in at least six directions to describe a voxel's diffusion tensor; therefore, DTI is a specific type of mathematical modeling of the DWI datasets. DTI enables the mean diffusivity (MD) and fractional anisotropy (FA) values to be determined. MD is the total diffusivity of the tissue, and FA indicates the degree of directional limitation observed for water diffusion. Diffusion tractography maps of white matter tracts have high FA values because the axons in white matter preferentially limit diffusion along the axon's longitudinal axis [81]. In a study [81], a cutoff MD value of 0.97 was identified as the most effective factor for the differential diagnosis between MB and brainstem gliomas, which reached a sensitivity of 96% and, a specificity of 100%, with MB MD values being lower than brainstem gliomas; also, the FA values for MBs were significantly higher than those for brainstem gliomas.

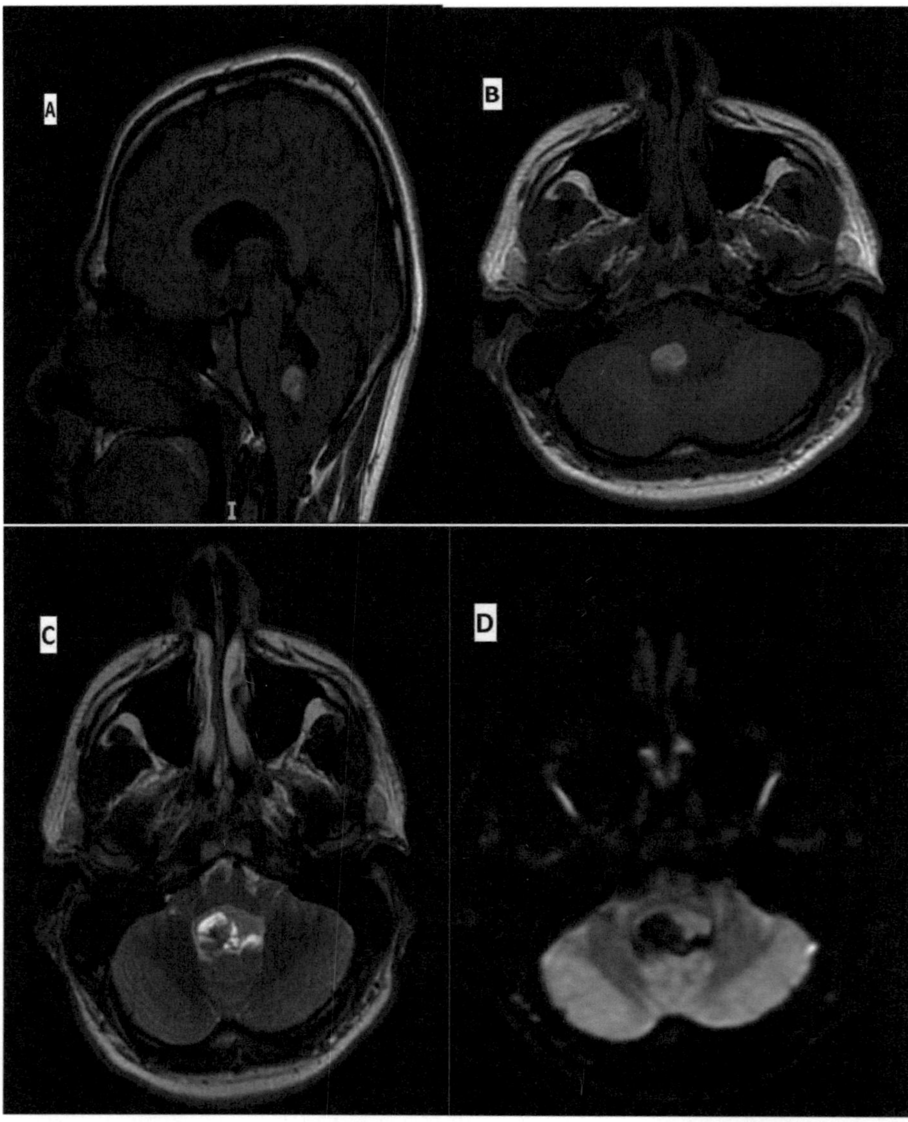

Figure 2.
Example of fourth ventricle ependymoma in a 23-year-old male arising from the floor of the fourth ventricle (the epicenter of the tumor is located inferior to the center of the fourth ventricle) (A). The mass is mixed solid and cystic, with the solid component appearing hypointense on T1 (B), mildly hyperintense on T2 (C), and the cystic component isointense on T1 (B) and hyperintense on T2 (C). The mass does not demonstrate restricted diffusion on the DWI scan (D).

MRS can be used to determine the metabolite profile from selected regions (voxels) of the tumor [36]. Hence, MRS can be used as a helpful tool to distinguish between the types of posterior fossa infiltrative brain tumors detected on MRI by detecting the presence of specific metabolic signals (e.g, N-acetylaspartate, choline, and lactate) and can also identify molecular subgroups within MB [7]. MB is associated with elevated taurine and choline with decreased N-acetylaspartate levels [74, 82, 83].

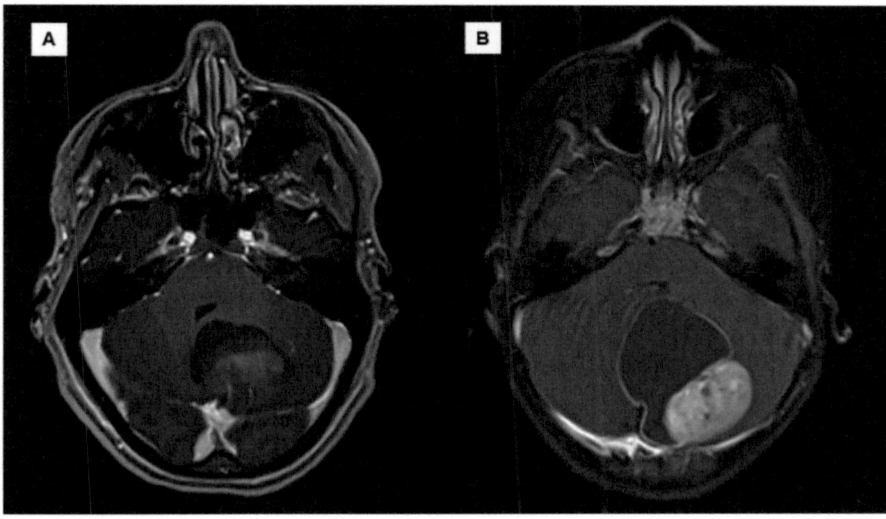

Figure 3.
Example of left cerebellar SHH-activated MB in a 24-year-old female (A). Classic pilocytic astrocytoma in a 4-year-old female with a mural contract-enhancing nodule in an enhancing cyst (B).

A 5-metabolite signature profile on MRS reliably differentiates SHH subgroup from non-WNT/non-SHH MB [84].

DWI is a quantitative MRI technique that provides spatial information on the random motion of water molecules in tissue (Brownian motion), combining intra-, trans-, and extracellular diffusion as well as perfusion [85]. It can be utilized to generate a signal contrast based on the differences in Brownian motion. High-grade tumors generally appear hyperintense on a DWI due to restrictions in water motion as they exhibit higher cellularity, tissue disorganization, and decreased extracellular space. The apparent diffusion coefficient (ADC) is a quantitative value that can be obtained from DWI and describes the magnitude of the motion of the water molecules independent of the direction. There is a strong inverse relationship between ADC and the density of tumorous tissue cells [86]. MB tumors appear bright on DWI and dark on corresponding ADC maps. Optimum threshold values of mean ADC extracted from solid portions of the tumor (i.e., solid only, not necrotic, cystic, or hemorrhagic components) can be used for differentiating tumor types [87–97]. When considering the mean ADC threshold values between MB and ependymoma, a meta-analysis performed by Dury et al. [98] reported a threshold value of 0.96 $mm^2/sec\ x10^{-3}$; lower values correlated more with medulloblastoma and higher values (1.26 $mm^2/sec \times 10^{-3}$) correlated more with ependymoma and pilocytic astrocytoma [44, 99]. Nonetheless, mean ADC values should be used in conjunction with other imaging features and clinical parameters to solidify the most likely diagnosis prior to obtaining a final pathology specimen. However, non-MB embryonal tumors such as AT/RT and ETMR cannot be reliably differentiated from MB as they have similar ADC values [45, 73].

Radiogenomics, as discussed previously, aims to define relationships between noninvasive imaging features and genomic data/molecular markers (molecular phenotypes). Imaging features such as size, margins, intensity, contrast enhancement, edema, necrosis, hemorrhage, and calcification can be assessed and quantified visually for correlation with molecular markers either singly or in combination. Computer-based algorithms supported by AI and machine learning approaches have refined the evaluation of many visual and mathematically defined imaging features [7].

Zhang and colleagues [100] conducted a retrospective study with seven institutions, including a total of 48 ATRTs and 96 patients with MB. They were able to identify six quantitative signatures of image intensity, texture, and morphology to distinguish ATRT from MB with high prediction performance. Among those, T2WI-based voxel intensities were most relevant. For example, the 90th percentile voxel intensity emerged as the most important predictive variable, with a higher value associated with ATRT. The myxoid background of the gelatinous mucopolysaccharide-rich water content that ATRT is known to produce contributes to the high T2-voxel intensity. In addition, heterogeneous texture predicts ATRT. The more heterogeneous texture of ATRT likely reflects multiple histologic components of rhabdoid cells juxtaposed to embryonal cells and sometimes glial and mesenchymal cells, compared with homogeneous and classically dense cellular sheet-pattern growth of MB. Most interestingly, linear and planar morphology suggested ATRT, whereas more circular and spherical morphology suggested MB (**Figure 4**).

In addition, radiogenomics allows preoperative identification of MB molecular subgroups based on multiparametric MRI, which is also an area of active research with promising early results [101–108]. Zhang and colleagues [109] performed a retrospective study at 12 international pediatric sites, with a total of 263 patients with MB, and developed a two-stage radiomics classifier that achieved an F1 core (measure of accuracy) of 88%, which can be used to infer the different molecular subgroups in a more accurate form. They identified that with T1-correlation, a global measure of homogeneity is greater for SHH but lower for the WNT group MB, as WNT exhibits more of a heterogeneous contrast enhancement compared to SHH. WNT tumors manifest vascular fragility with blood-brain barrier breakdown, which might also render tumor intensities more heterogeneous [110].

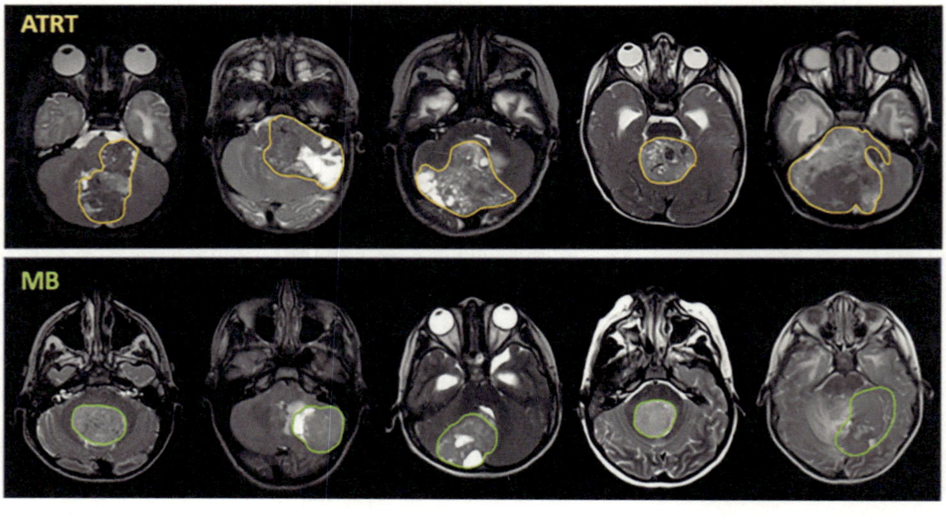

Figure 4.
MR imaging correlates of radiomics phenotypes to distinguish between ATRT and MB. More heterogeneous features correlated with ATRT. Spheric morphology correlated with MB as compared with the more elongated or planar configuration of ATRT.

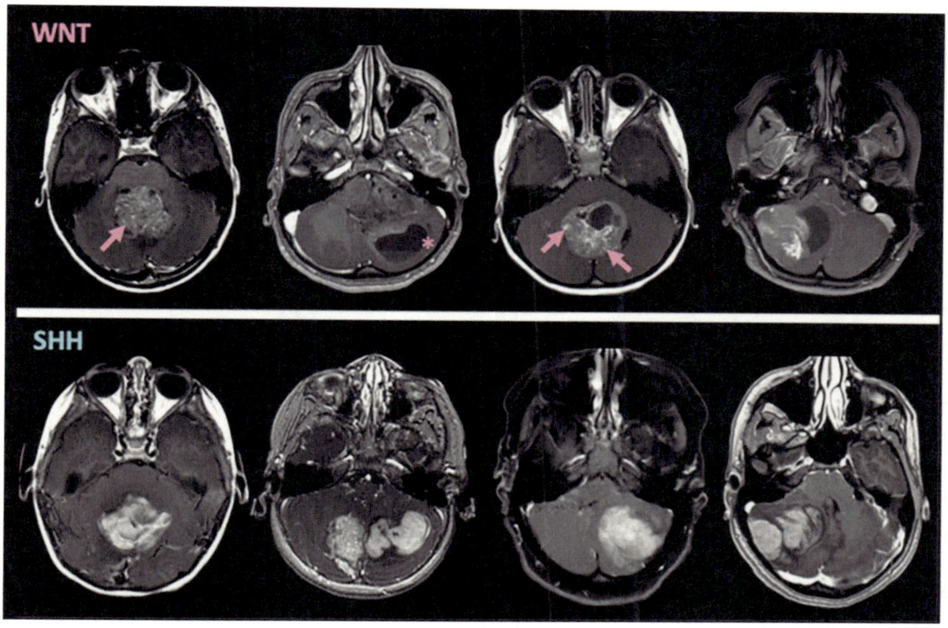

Figure 5.
MR imaging correlates radiomics phenotypes to distinguish between SHH and WNT MB. More heterogeneous features correlated with WNT compared to SHH.

Preoperative image phenotypes predictive of WNT could potentially offer a surgeon the option of less invasive or lower-risk surgery. This can have clinical implications as lesions that lateralize to the cerebellar peduncle, and thus are at a higher risk for mutism, may benefit from a biopsy, as WNT tumors may respond better to chemo-RT alone (**Figure 5**).

7. Current role of postoperative imaging

Treatment paradigms for MB include multimodality therapy consisting of surgery followed by adjuvant RT and systemic chemotherapy. The standard neurosurgical procedure is maximal safe resection. Following maximal safe resection of the tumor, MRI is needed to assess the extent of resection and quantify residual tumor for assigning risk [111] and hence determine further adjuvant therapy. Ideally, postoperative MRI is performed within 24–48 hours of surgical resection. Delays beyond that make it difficult to detect and interpret residual tumors due to blood and blood products present in the resection cavity, as well as postsurgical enhancing reactive gliosis can complicate the detection of residual disease [7, 70]. If MRI was obtained beyond the 24–48 hour window when extensive parenchymal postoperative changes might be obscuring a residual tumor or enhancing reactive gliosis might be falsely regarded as a residual tumor, RAPNO guidelines recommend obtaining a second MRI 2–3 weeks after surgery to better assess the extent of resection and allow some time for the postoperative changes to resolve [70, 75]. The presence or absence of residual disease directly affects protocol assignment in clinical trials.

In patients without a preoperative spinal MRI, the spine should be imaged either within 24–48 hours of surgery (at the time of brain imaging) or 2–3 weeks after to avoid false positive results arising from postoperative leptomeningeal enhancement and subdural collections [70, 75]. Postoperative MRI is also helpful in identifying postsurgical complications such as posterior fossa/cerebellar mutism, hemorrhage, meningitis, pseudomeningocele, and cervical spine instability. Mutism syndrome after posterior fossa tumor surgery has been reported to be variable (ranging from 8 to 39%) [112]. Symptoms can present as reduced speech, emotional lability, hypotonia, apraxia, ataxia, and cognitive impairment. Patients can develop mutism immediately or 1–7 days after surgery. Commonly, mutism lasts for 1–3 months after surgery [113]. Residual sequelae with long-term linguistic impairments such as low speech speed, dysarthria, and motor impairment are seen in a small proportion of patients. Although the etiology remains unclear, the most prevalent hypothesis is that cerebro-cerebellar diaschisis plays a crucial role in mutism development. Several studies have identified certain imaging features such as a large tumor (size > = 5 cm), tumor infiltration into the brainstem, attachment to the floor of the fourth ventricle, and periventricular ischemia as protentional risk factors for developing mutism syndrome [114].

Postoperative adjuvant treatment in MB has been generally based on a clinical radiological risk stratification system [111], where patients over the age of three at initial diagnosis with postoperative residual tumor <1.5 cm^2 (R0) and without metastasis were classified as having average-risk disease. High-risk disease was defined as the presence of any one of the following features; < 3 years, residual tumor > = 1.5 cm^2 (R+), and any evidence of metastasis (M+). Postoperative adjuvant RT and systemic chemotherapy are the cornerstones of curative intent treatment for MB [7].

8. Current role of imaging for RT treatment planning

RT forms an integral component of the management paradigm for MB. With more children achieving long-term survival after therapy, late effects of RT, including neurocognitive damage, growth arrest, and second cancers, have become an important concern. Recent advances in image-guided capabilities and RT delivery technologies such as proton therapy have led to a new era of precision treatment with significantly less exposure to healthy tissues.

RT target volumes encompass the entire neuroaxis, i.e., craniospinal irradiation (CSI), which is the whole brain, entire meningeal reflections, complete spinal canal, and thecal sac, followed by boost irradiation of the tumor bed to achieve adequate disease control.

Therapeutic adjuvant RT needs to begin promptly, typically within 4 weeks of surgery, once the patient recovers postoperatively. The CSI dose prescribed is dependent on accurately defining risk and other factors. In average-risk MB, reduced-dose CSI (23.4 Gy) plus tumor bed boost (30.6 Gy) along with adjuvant multiagent systemic chemotherapy results in excellent long-term survival outcomes and reduced neurocognitive and endocrinologic sequelae compared to higher-dose CSI (36 Gy) [7]. If chemotherapy is not available or deemed unacceptable, the CSI dose is 36 Gy plus a tumor bed boost of 18–19.8 Gy can be offered with equal efficacy. For high-risk MB, the standard CSI dose is 36 Gy, and a tumor bed boost of 18–19.8 Gy. Generally, it is recommended that the dose for the primary tumor be 54–55.8 Gy delivered over 6 weeks using conventional fractionation. Selected patients with diffuse leptomeningeal dissemination may be treated with extended-dose CSI (39.6–40 Gy) plus treatment to the entire posterior fossa to a boost dose of 14.4 Gy. An additional boost of 5.4–9 Gy to focal nodular metastatic deposits in the brain and/or spine can be delivered concurrently during posterior fossa boost RT.

RT may be delivered with high-energy photons (X-rays created by a medical linear accelerator) or protons produced in a cyclotron or synchrotron. Both techniques have evolved to diminish the RT dose to normal tissues and hence diminish both acute and late toxicities.

9. Image-guided RT

Adaptive RT aims to customize each patient's daily treatment plan to the known patient-specific variation (whether anatomical or positional set-ups) and hence optimize the dose delivered both to the tumor and surrounding normal tissues. Image-guided RT has become widely available in recent years. Many RT treatment units (both photon and proton) are now equipped to take high-quality images with CT with the patient in the treatment position before RT is delivered. Images can be kvCBCT (cone beam computed tomography), a form of advanced medical imaging that utilizes kV X-rays with high contrast, unlike traditional megavoltage CT. CBCT uses divergent X-rays, creating a cone-shaped beam by utilizing diagnostic (kV) X-rays to the target area to provide images with higher contrast. MRI-guided RT has more recently become available and provides superior soft-tissue contrast, organ motion visualization, and the ability to monitor tumor and tissue physiologic changes. However, it is currently only available with photons.

The most commonly used image for CSI image guidance is the CT scan, due to its superior bony landmarks visualization, which is used to identify the correct position and alignment for CSI treatments; however, in the subsequent boost treatments used in standard-risk MB, MRI-guided therapy is preferred due to its superior soft-tissue contrast, allowing for a better visualization of the tumor bed cavity and/or the residual tumor itself if present.

10. Current role of imaging in follow-up and surveillance

The main objective of imaging during follow-up is the detection of early recurrences. However, whether detecting asymptomatic recurrences on surveillance imaging leads to improved survival or just reflects lead time bias is unclear. The data regarding this has been conflicting with contradictory results from previous studies [115–117], justifying prospective studies to explore the benefit and most favorable timing of follow-up surveillance MRI.

Most guidelines recommend MRI scans in the initial 2–3 years following treatment once every 3 months. After 3 years the frequency can be extended to once every 6 months until 5 years followed by yearly MRIs. The differences in the incidence, pattern, and time to first relapse among the molecular subgroups are becoming evident [118–120]. This may affect the frequency of future surveillance imaging. The role of follow-up MRI of the spine has been doubtful. Bartels et al. [121] reported no isolated spinal recurrences (without intracranial recurrence) in a cohort of 73 children with MB followed by surveillance brain and spine MRI [7], suggesting that MRI of the spine may not be necessary in patients with low- or standard-risk disease provided there is no demonstrable recurrence within the first 2 years after completing therapy. For patients with high-risk disease, it is recommended to obtain a spine MRI every

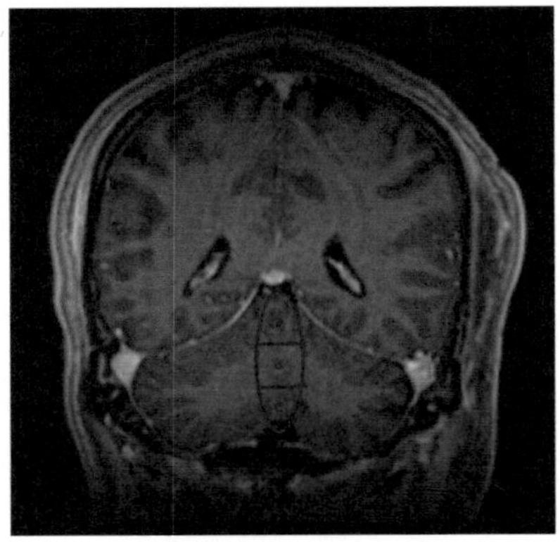

Figure 6.
Coronal MRI-T2W demonstrating the three subsites of the vermis (upper, middle, and lower).

3 months in the first 2 years, then annually for the following 3 years, if clinically indicated. Patients with new-onset neurological symptoms or worsening existing symptoms should raise suspicion for disease recurrence, mandating an urgent MRI. For patients with evidence of disease recurrence in the brain, complete neuroaxis staging should be considered to assess overall tumor burden and multimodality salvage treatment strategy.

DWI has been shown to be more effective than conventional MRI in recent studies to detect early recurrences and differentiate them from treatment-related changes [122, 123]. In a study by Aboian et al. evaluating 21 pediatric patients with definitive recurrent disease in the brain, MRIs at diagnosis of recurrence and 6 months prior were evaluated for new lesions with reduced diffusion on DWI, contrast enhancement, size, and location of recurrence. All recurrent MB lesions demonstrated reduced diffusion. Apparent diffusion coefficient (ADC) measurements were statistically significantly lower ($P = .00001$) in recurrent lesions as compared to the contralateral normal region of interest. Contrast enhancement within the recurrent lesions was seen in sixteen patients (76.2%) with disease recurrence. All five patients with non-enhancing recurrence showed reduced diffusion, with a mean ADC of 0.695 ± 0.101 (normal = 0.893 ± 0.100, $P = .0027$) [123].

As survival improves, treatment-related toxicity challenges are seen that have the potential to significantly impact quality of life. The incidence, spectrum of onset, and severity of complications can vary, with mutism manifesting directly after surgery, endocrinopathies and neurocognitive dysfunction presenting some years post therapy, and secondary malignancies or cerebrovascular accidents presenting after decades. While surveillance imaging has focused on detecting recurrent disease, continuing research is targeting the timely detection and prediction of late complications. It has been established that young age (i.e., less than 7 years) and higher doses of CSI are clinical predictors of a higher risk of neurocognitive decline [122, 123]. However, localization and size of the tumor are radiological risk factors for reduced cognition with RT as well [124, 125].

Józefacka et al. [126] studied imaging findings in 13 pediatric medulloblastoma patients after 3 years or more since their treatment completion. Two discriminative factors were identified as being associated with lower cognitive performance of the survivors: tumor extending to the foramen of Luschka and excision of the middle part of the vermis (**Figure 6**).

11. Conclusion

Imaging plays a critical role in all aspects of the management of patients with MB. The initial diagnosis, staging, RT treatment planning, and follow-up all require high-quality neuroimaging that is increasingly complex and informative. Working in a multi-disciplinary environment with experts in neuroradiology is essential.

Conflict of interest

The authors declare no conflict of interest.

Author details

Hebah Abudawaba[1], Vinaya Rajahraman[2], Maryann Bishop-Jodoin[2] and John M. Buatti[1]*

1 Department of Radiation Oncology, The University of Iowa, Iowa City, IA, USA

2 Department of Radiation Oncology, University of Massachusetts Chan Medical School, Worcester, MA, USA

*Address all correspondence to: john-buatti@uiowa.edu

References

[1] Ostrom QT, Price M, Neff C, Cioffi G, Waite KA, Kruchko C, et al. CBTRUS statistical report: Primary brain and other central nervous system Tumors diagnosed in the United States in 2015-2019. Neuro-Oncology. 2022;**24**(S5):v1-v95. DOI: 10.1093/neuonc/noac202

[2] McKean-Cowdin R, Razavi P, Barrington-Trimis J, Baldwin RT, Asgharzadeh S, Cockburn M, et al. Trends in childhood brain tumor incidence, 1973-2009. Journal of Neuro-Oncology. 2013;**115**(2):153-160. DOI: 10.1007/s11060-013-1212-5

[3] Ostrom QT, Gittleman H, Fulop J, Liu M, Blanda R, Kromer C, et al. CBTRUS statistical report: Primary brain and central nervous system tumors diagnosed in the United States in 2008-2012. Neuro-Oncology. 2015;**17**(S4):iv1-iv62. DOI: 10.1093/neuonc/nov189

[4] Brandes AA, Bartolotti M, Marucci G, Ghimenton C, Agati R, Fioravanti A, et al. New perspectives in the treatment of adult medulloblastoma in the era of molecular oncology. Critical Reviews in Oncology/Hematology. 2015;**94**(3):348-359. DOI: 10.1016/j.critrevonc.2014.12.016

[5] Louis DN, Ohgaki H, Wiestler OD, Cavenee WK, Burger PC, et al. The 2007 WHO classification of tumours of the central nervous system. Acta Neuropathologica. 2007;**114**(2):97-109. DOI: 10.1007/s00401-007-0243-4

[6] Louis DN, Perry A, Reifenberger G, von Deimling A, Figarella-Branger D, Cavenee WK, et al. The 2016 World Health Organization classification of tumors of the central nervous system: A summary. Acta Neuropathologica. 2016;**131**(6):803-820. DOI: 10.1007/s00401-016-1545-1

[7] Dasgupta A, Maitre M, Pungavkar S, Gupta T. Magnetic resonance imaging in the contemporary management of medulloblastoma: Current and emerging applications. Methods in Molecular Biology. 2022;**2423**:187-214. DOI: 10.1007/978-1-0716-1952-0_18

[8] Mechtler L. Neuroimaging in neuro-oncology. Neurologic Clinics. 2009;**27**(1):171-201, ix. DOI: 10.1016/j.ncl.2008.09.015

[9] Bradley WG. History of medical imaging. Proceedings of the American Philosophical Society. 2008;**152**(3):349-361

[10] Castillo M. History and evolution of brain tumor imaging: Insights through radiology. Radiology. 2014;**273**(S2):S111-S125. DOI: 10.1148/radiol.14140130

[11] Scatliff JH, Morris PJ. From roentgen to magnetic resonance imaging: The history of medical imaging. North Carolina Medical Journal. 2014;**75**(2):111-113. DOI: 10.18043/ncm.75.2.111

[12] Hoeffner EG, Mukherji SK, Srinivasan A, Quint DJ. Neuroradiology back to the future: Brain imaging. AJNR. American Journal of Neuroradiology. 2012;**33**(1):5-11. DOI: 10.3174/ajnr.A2936

[13] Lutters B, Koehler PJ. Cerebral pneumography and the 20th century localization of brain tumours. Brain. 2018;**141**(3):927-933. DOI: 10.1093/brain/awy031

[14] Doby T. Cerebral angiography and Egas Moniz. AJR. American Journal

of Roentgenology. 1992;**159**(2):364. DOI: 10.2214/ajr.159.2.1632357

[15] Bull JW. The history of neuroradiology. Proceedings of the Royal Society of Medicine. 1970;**63**(6):637-643

[16] Leeds NE, Goldberg HI. Abnormal vascular patterns in benign intracranial lesions: Pseudotumors of the brain. The American Journal of Roentgenology, Radium Therapy, and Nuclear Medicine. 1973;**118**(3):576-585. DOI: 10.2214/ajr.118.3.576

[17] List CF, Hodges FJ. Differential diagnosis of intracranial neoplasms by cerebral angiography. Radiology. 1947;**48**(5):493-508. DOI: 10.1148/48.5.493

[18] Pietrzak A, Marszałek A, Piotrowski T, Pietrasz K, Medak A, Wojtowicz J, et al. The utility of ^{18}F-FDG PET/CT in brain tumours diagnosis. Reports of Practical Oncology and Radiotherapy. 2022;**27**(2):235-240. DOI: 10.5603/RPOR.a2022.0021

[19] Verger A, Kas A, Darcourt J, Guedj E. PET imaging in neuro-oncology: An update and overview of a rapidly growing area. Cancers (Basel). 2022;**14**(5):1103. DOI: 10.3390/cancers14051103

[20] Hounsfield GN. Computerized transverse axial scanning (tomography). 1. Description of system. The British Journal of Radiology. 1973;**46**(552):1016-1022. DOI: 10.1259/0007-1285-46-552-1016

[21] Ambrose J. Computerized transverse axial scanning (tomography). 2. Clinical application. The British Journal of Radiology. 1973;**46**(552):1023-1047. DOI: 10.1259/0007-1285-46-552-1023

[22] Hoeffner EG, Mukherji SK, Srinivasan A, Quint DJ. Neuroradiology back to the future: Spine imaging. AJNR. American Journal of Neuroradiology. 2012;**33**(6):999-1006. DOI: 10.3174/ajnr.A3129

[23] Schulz RA, Stein JA, Pelc NJ. How CT happened: The early development of medical computed tomography. Journal of Medical Imaging (Bellingham). 2021;**8**(5):052110. DOI: 10.1117/1.JMI.8.5.052110

[24] Amundsen P, Dugstad G, Noyes W. Cerebral angiography via the femoral artery with particular reference to cerebrovascular disease. Acta Neurologica Scandinavica. 1967;**43**(S31):115. DOI: 10.1111/j.1600-0404.1967.tb02073.x

[25] Bull J. Editorial: The changing face of neuroradiology over nearly forty years. Neuroradiology. 1975;**9**(3):111-115. DOI: 10.1007/BF00332956

[26] Huckman MS. Neuroradiology without benefit of computers: A memoir. AJNR. American Journal of Neuroradiology. 2010;**31**(5):784-786. DOI: 10.3174/ajnr.A1935

[27] Damadian R. Tumor detection by nuclear magnetic resonance. Science. 1971;**171**(3976):1151-1153. DOI: 10.1126/science.171.3976.1151

[28] Lauterbur PC. Image formation by induced local interactions. Examples employing nuclear magnetic resonance 1973. Clinical Orthopaedics and Related Research. 1989;(244):3-6

[29] Rosenbaum AE et al. In re: Amundsen P. Cerebral angiography via the femoral artery with particular reference to cerebrovascular disease. Acta Neurol Scand 1967; Suppl. 31:115. AJNR. American Journal of Neuroradiology. 2001;**22**(3):584-589

[30] Kim PE, Zee CS. Imaging of the cerebrum. Neurosurgery. 2007;**61**(1S): 123-146; discussion 146. DOI: 10.1227/01.neu.0000279316.03266.cd

[31] Zoarski GH, Lufkin RB, Bradley WG Jr, Flanders AE, Gale DR, Harms SE, et al. Multicenter trial of gadoteridol, a nonionic gadolinium chelate, in patients with suspected head and neck pathology. AJNR. American Journal of Neuroradiology. 1993;**14**(4):955-961

[32] Hoeffner EG, Mukherji SK, Srinivasan A, Quint DJ. Neuroradiology back to the future: Head and neck imaging. AJNR. American Journal of Neuroradiology. 2012;**33**(11):2026-2032. DOI: 10.3174/ajnr.A3365

[33] Runge VM, Carollo BR, Wolf CR, Nelson KL, Gelblum DY. Gd DTPA: A review of clinical indications in central nervous system magnetic resonance imaging. Radiographics. 1989;**9**(5):929-958. DOI: 10.1148/radiographics.9.5.2678298

[34] Purandare NC. Inclusion of brain in FDG PET/CT scanning techniques in cancer patients: Does it obviate the need for dedicated brain imaging? Indian Journal of Nuclear Medicine. 2011;**26**(2):64-66. DOI: 10.4103/0972-3919.90253

[35] Raslan O, Ozturk A, Oguz KK, Sen F, Aboud O, Ivanovic V, et al. Imaging cancer in neuroradiology. Current Problems in Cancer. 2023;**47**(2):100965. DOI: 10.1016/j.currproblcancer.2023.100965

[36] Villanueva-Meyer JE, Mabray MC, Cha S. Current clinical brain tumor imaging. Neurosurgery. 2017;**81**(3):397-415. DOI: 10.1093/neuros/nyx103

[37] Cha S. Update on brain tumor imaging. Current Neurology and Neuroscience Reports. 2005;**5**(3):169-177. DOI: 10.1007/s11910-005-0044-x

[38] Ellingson BM, Bendszus M, Boxerman J, Barboriak D, Erickson BJ, Smits M, et al. Consensus recommendations for a standardized brain tumor imaging protocol in clinical trials. Neuro-Oncology. 2015;**17**(9):1188-1198. DOI: 10.1093/neuonc/nov095

[39] Wamelink IJHG, Azizova A, Booth TC, Mutsaerts HJMM, Ogunleye A, Mankad K, et al. Brain tumor imaging without gadolinium-based contrast agents: Feasible or fantasy? Radiology. 2024;**310**(2):e230793. DOI: 10.1148/radiol.230793

[40] Nag S, Manias JL, Stewart DJ. Pathology and new players in the pathogenesis of brain edema. Acta Neuropathologica. 2009;**118**(2):197-217. DOI: 10.1007/s00401-009-0541-0

[41] Stummer W. Mechanisms of tumor-related brain edema. Neurosurgical Focus. 2007;**22**(5):E8. DOI: 10.3171/foc.2007.22.5.9

[42] Gaddamanugu S, Shafaat O, Sotoudeh H, Sarrami AH, Rezaei A, Saadatpour Z, et al. Clinical applications of diffusion-weighted sequence in brain imaging: Beyond stroke. Neuroradiology. 2022;**64**(1):15-30. DOI: 10.1007/s00234-021-02819-3

[43] Romano A, Palizzi S, Romano A, Moltoni G, Di Napoli A, Maccioni F, et al. Diffusion weighted imaging in neuro-oncology: Diagnosis, post-treatment changes, and advanced sequences-an updated review. Cancers (Basel). 2023;**15**(3):618. DOI: 10.3390/cancers15030618

[44] Pierce T, Kranz PG, Roth C, Leong D, Wei P, Provenzale JM. Use of apparent diffusion coefficient values for diagnosis

of pediatric posterior fossa tumors. The Neuroradiology Journal. 2014;**27**(2):233-244. DOI: 10.15274/NRJ-2014-10027

[45] Yamashita Y, Kumabe T, Higano S, Watanabe M, Tominaga T. Minimum apparent diffusion coefficient is significantly correlated with cellularity in medulloblastomas. Neurological Research. 2009;**31**(9):940-946. DOI: 10.1179/174313209X382520

[46] Essig M, Nguyen TB, Shiroishi MS, Saake M, Provenzale JM, wt al. Perfusion MRI: The five most frequently asked clinical questions. AJR. American Journal of Roentgenology. 2013;**201**(3):W495-W510. DOI: 10.2214/AJR.12.9544

[47] Gharzeddine K, Hatzoglou V, Holodny AI, Young RJ. MR perfusion and MR spectroscopy of brain neoplasms. Radiologic Clinics of North America. 2019;**57**(6):1177-1188. DOI: 10.1016/j.rcl.2019.07.008

[48] Lin A, Tran T, Bluml S, Merugumala S, Liao HJ, Ross BD. Guidelines for acquiring and reporting clinical neurospectroscopy. Seminars in Neurology. 2012;**32**(4):432-453. DOI: 10.1055/s-0032-1331814

[49] Shahar T, Rozovski U, Marko NF, Tummala S, Ziu M, Weinberg JS, et al. Preoperative imaging to predict intraoperative changes in tumor-to-corticospinal tract distance: An analysis of 45 cases using high-field intraoperative magnetic resonance imaging. Neurosurgery. 2014;**75**(1):23-30. DOI: 10.1227/NEU.0000000000000338

[50] Wang L, Chen D, Olson J, Ali S, Fan T, Mao H. Re-examine tumor-induced alterations in hemodynamic responses of BOLD fMRI: Implications in presurgical brain mapping. Acta Radiologica. 2012;**53**(7):802-811. DOI: 10.1258/ar.2012.120118

[51] van Timmeren JE, Cester D, Tanadini-Lang S, Alkadhi H, Baessler B. Radiomics in medical imaging-"how-to" guide and critical reflection. Insights into Imaging. 2020;**11**(1):91. DOI: 10.1186/s13244-020-00887-2

[52] Castellano G, Bonilha L, Li LM, Cendes F. Texture analysis of medical images. Clinical Radiology. 2004;**59**(12):1061-1069. DOI: 10.1016/j.crad.2004.07.008

[53] Mannil M, von Spiczak J, Manka R, Alkadhi H. Texture analysis and machine learning for detecting myocardial infarction in noncontrast low-dose computed tomography: Unveiling the invisible. Investigative Radiology. 2018;**53**(6):338-343. DOI: 10.1097/RLI.0000000000000448

[54] Lohmann P, Bousabarah K, Hoevels M, Treuer H. Radiomics in radiation oncology-basics, methods, and limitations. Strahlentherapie und Onkologie. 2020;**196**(10):848-855. DOI: 10.1007/s00066-020-01663-3

[55] Zwanenburg A, Vallières M, Abdalah MA, Aerts HJWL, Andrearczyk V, Apte A, et al. The image biomarker standardization initiative: Standardized quantitative radiomics for high-throughput image-based phenotyping. Radiology. 2020;**295**(2):328-338. DOI: 10.1148/radiol.2020191145

[56] Forghani R. Precision digital oncology: Emerging role of radiomics-based biomarkers and artificial intelligence for advanced imaging and characterization of brain tumors. Radiology: Imaging Cancer. 2020;**2**(4):e190047. DOI: 10.1148/rycan.2020190047

[57] Artzi M, Bressler I, Ben BD. Differentiation between glioblastoma, brain metastasis and subtypes using radiomics analysis. Journal of Magnetic Resonance Imaging. 2019;**50**(2):519-528. DOI: 10.1002/jmri.26643

[58] Sengupta A, Agarwal S, Gupta PK, Ahlawat S, Patir R, Gupta RK, et al. On differentiation between vasogenic edema and non-enhancing tumor in high-grade glioma patients using a support vector machine classifier based upon pre and post-surgery MRI images. European Journal of Radiology. 2018;**106**:199-208. DOI: 10.1016/j.ejrad.2018.07.018

[59] Su C, Jiang J, Zhang S, Shi J, Xu K, Shen N, et al. Radiomics based on multicontrast MRI can precisely differentiate among glioma subtypes and predict tumour-proliferative behaviour. European Radiology. 2019;**29**(4):1986-1996. DOI: 10.1007/s00330-018-5704-8

[60] Li Y, Qian Z, Xu K, Wang K, Fan X, Li S, et al. MRI features predict p53 status in lower-grade gliomas via a machine-learning approach. NeuroImage Clinical. 2018;**17**:306-311. DOI: 10.1016/j.nicl.2017.10.030

[61] Laukamp KR, Thiele F, Shakirin G, Zopfs D, Faymonville A, Timmer M, et al. Fully automated detection and segmentation of meningiomas using deep learning on routine multiparametric MRI. European Radiology. 2019;**29**(1):124-132. DOI: 10.1007/s00330-018-5595-8

[62] Peng L, Parekh V, Huang P, Lin DD, Sheikh K, Baker B, et al. Distinguishing true progression from radionecrosis after stereotactic radiation therapy for brain metastases with machine learning and radiomics. International Journal of Radiation Oncology, Biology, Physics. 2018;**102**(4):1236-1243. DOI: 10.1016/j.ijrobp.2018.05.041

[63] Koeller KK, Rushing EJ. From the archives of the AFIP: Medulloblastoma: A comprehensive review with radiologic-pathologic correlation. Radiographics. 2003;**23**(6):1613-1637. DOI: 10.1148/rg.236035168

[64] Poretti A, Meoded A, Huisman TA. Neuroimaging of pediatric posterior fossa tumors including review of the literature. Journal of Magnetic Resonance Imaging. 2012;**35**(1):32-47. DOI: 10.1002/jmri.22722

[65] Rasalkar DD, Chu WC, Paunipagar BK, Cheng FW, Li CK. Paediatric intra-axial posterior fossa tumours: pictorial review. Postgraduate Medical Journal. 2013;**89**(1047):39-46. DOI: 10.1136/postgradmedj-2011-130075

[66] Chatterjee A, Maitre M, Dasgupta A, Srdhar E. Magnetic resonance imaging in the contemporary management of medulloblastoma: Current and emerging applications. In: Dey A, Malhotra A, Garg N, editors. Medulloblastoma. 1st ed. New York: Humana; 2022. p. 187-214. Chapter 19. DOI: 10.1007/978-1-0716-1952-0

[67] Dasgupta A, Gupta T, Pungavkar S, Shirsat N, Epari S, Chinnaswamy G, et al. Nomograms based on preoperative multiparametric magnetic resonance imaging for prediction of molecular subgrouping in medulloblastoma: Results from a radiogenomics study of 111 patients. Neuro-Oncology. 2019;**21**(1):115-124. DOI: 10.1093/neuonc/noy093

[68] Schweitzer T, Vince GH, Herbold C, Roosen K, Tonn JC. Extraneural metastases of primary brain tumors. Journal of Neuro-Oncology. 2001;**53**(2):107-114. DOI: 10.1023/a:1012245115209

[69] Gupta T, Dasgupta A, Epari S, Shirsat N, Chinnaswamy G,

Jalali R. Extraneuraxial metastases in medulloblastoma: Is histology and molecular biology important? Journal of Neuro-Oncology. 2017;**135**(2):419-421. DOI: 10.1007/s11060-017-2586-6

[70] Warren KE, Vezina G, Poussaint TY, Warmuth-Metz M, Chamberlain MC, Packer RJ, et al. Response assessment in medulloblastoma and leptomeningeal seeding tumors: Recommendations from the response assessment in Pediatric neuro-oncology committee. Neuro-Oncology. 2018;**20**(1):13-23. DOI: 10.1093/neuonc/nox087

[71] Fouladi M, Gajjar A, Boyett JM, Walter AW, Thompson SJ, Merchant TE, et al. Comparison of CSF cytology and spinal magnetic resonance imaging in the detection of leptomeningeal disease in pediatric medulloblastoma or primitive neuroectodermal tumor. Journal of Clinical Oncology. 1999;**17**(10):3234-3237. DOI: 10.1200/JCO.1999.17.10.3234

[72] Meyers SP, Khademian ZP, Biegel JA, Chuang SH, Korones DN, Zimmerman RA. Primary intracranial atypical teratoid/rhabdoid tumors of infancy and childhood: MRI features and patient outcomes. AJNR. American Journal of Neuroradiology. 2006;**27**(5):962-971

[73] Koral K, Gargan L, Bowers DC, Gimi B, Timmons CF, Weprin B, et al. Imaging characteristics of atypical teratoid-rhabdoid tumor in children compared with medulloblastoma. AJR. American Journal of Roentgenology. 2008;**190**(3):809-814. DOI: 10.2214/AJR.07.3069

[74] Fruehwald-Pallamar J, Puchner SB, Rossi A, Garre ML, Cama A, Koelblinger C, et al. Magnetic resonance imaging spectrum of medulloblastoma. Neuroradiology. 2011;**53**(6):387-396. DOI: 10.1007/s00234-010-0829-8

[75] Yeom KW, Mobley BC, Lober RM, Andre JB, Partap S, Vogel H, et al. Distinctive MRI features of pediatric medulloblastoma subtypes. AJR. American Journal of Roentgenology. 2013;**200**(4):895-903. DOI: 10.2214/AJR.12.9249

[76] Teo WY, Shen J, Su JM, Yu A, Wang J, Chow WY, et al. Implications of tumor location on subtypes of medulloblastoma. Pediatric Blood & Cancer. 2013;**60**(9):1408-1410. DOI: 10.1002/pbc.24511

[77] Wefers AK, Warmuth-Metz M, Pöschl J, von Bueren AO, Monoranu CM, Seelos K, et al. Subgroup-specific localization of human medulloblastoma based on pre-operative MRI. Acta Neuropathologica. 2014;**127**(6):931-933. DOI: 10.1007/s00401-014-1271-5

[78] Dasgupta A, Gupta T, Sridhar E, Shirsat N, Krishnatry R, Goda JS, et al. Pediatric patients with SHH medulloblastoma fail differently as compared with adults: Possible implications for treatment modifications. Journal of Pediatric Hematology/Oncology. 2019;**41**(8):e499-e505. DOI: 10.1097/MPH.0000000000001484

[79] Brandão LA, Young PT. Posterior fossa tumors. Neuroimaging Clinics of North America. 2017;**27**(1):1-37. DOI: 10.1016/j.nic.2016.08.001

[80] Chourmouzi D, Papadopoulou E, Konstantinidis M, Syrris V, Kouskouras K, Haritanti A, et al. Manifestations of pilocytic astrocytoma: A pictorial review. Insights into Imaging. 2014;**5**(3):387-402. DOI: 10.1007/s13244-014-0328-2

[81] Duc NM. The role of diffusion tensor imaging metrics in the discrimination between cerebellar medulloblastoma and brainstem glioma. Pediatric

Blood & Cancer. 2020;**67**(9):e28468. DOI: 10.1002/pbc.28468

[82] Kovanlikaya A, Panigrahy A, Krieger MD, Gonzalez-Gomez I, Ghugre N, McComb JG, et al. Untreated pediatric primitive neuroectodermal tumor in vivo: Quantitation of taurine with MR spectroscopy. Radiology. 2005;**236**(3):1020-1025. DOI: 10.1148/radiol.2363040856

[83] Panigrahy A, Krieger MD, Gonzalez-Gomez I, Liu X, McComb JG, Finlay JL, et al. Quantitative short echo time 1H-MR spectroscopy of untreated pediatric brain tumors: Preoperative diagnosis and characterization. AJNR. American Journal of Neuroradiology. 2006;**27**(3):560-572

[84] Blüml S, Margol AS, Sposto R, Kennedy RJ, Robison NJ, Vali M, et al. Molecular subgroups of medulloblastoma identification using noninvasive magnetic resonance spectroscopy. Neuro-Oncology. 2016;**18**(1):126-131. DOI: 10.1093/neuonc/nov097

[85] Hagmann P, Jonasson L, Maeder P, Thiran JP, Wedeen VJ, Meuli R. Understanding diffusion MR imaging techniques: From scalar diffusion-weighted imaging to diffusion tensor imaging and beyond. Radiographics. 2006;**26**(S1):S205-S223. DOI: 10.1148/rg.26si065510

[86] Surov A, Meyer HJ, Wienke A. Correlation between apparent diffusion coefficient (ADC) and cellularity is different in several tumors: A meta-analysis. Oncotarget. 2017;**8**(35):59492-59499. DOI: 10.18632/oncotarget.17752

[87] Assis ZA, Saini J, Ranjan M, Gupta AK, Sabharwal P, Naidu PR. Diffusion tensor imaging in evaluation of posterior fossa tumors in children on a 3T MRI scanner. Indian Journal of Radiology and Imaging. 2015;**25**(4):445-452. DOI: 10.4103/0971-3026.169444

[88] Bull JG, Saunders DE, Clark CA. Discrimination of paediatric brain tumours using apparent diffusion coefficient histograms. European Radiology. 2012;**22**(2):447-457. DOI: 10.1007/s00330-011-2255-7

[89] Domínguez-Pinilla N, Martínez de Aragón A, Diéguez Tapias S, Toldos O, Hinojosa Bernal J, Rigal Andrés M, et al. Evaluating the apparent diffusion coefficient in MRI studies as a means of determining paediatric brain tumour stages. Neurología. 2016;**31**(7):459-465. DOI: 10.1016/j.nrl.2014.12.003

[90] Gauvain KM, McKinstry RC, Mukherjee P, Perry A, Neil JJ, Kaufman BA, et al. Evaluating pediatric brain tumor cellularity with diffusion-tensor imaging. AJR. American Journal of Roentgenology. 2001;**177**(2):449-454. DOI: 10.2214/ajr.177.2.1770449

[91] Gimi B, Cederberg K, Derinkuyu B, Gargan L, Koral KM, Bowers DC, et al. Utility of apparent diffusion coefficient ratios in distinguishing common pediatric cerebellar tumors. Academic Radiology. 2012;**19**(7):794-800. DOI: 10.1016/j.acra.2012.03.004

[92] Koral K, Alford R, Choudhury N, Mossa-Basha M, Gargan L, Gimi B, et al. Applicability of apparent diffusion coefficient ratios in preoperative diagnosis of common pediatric cerebellar tumors across two institutions. Neuroradiology. 2014;**56**(9):781-788. DOI: 10.1007/s00234-014-1398-z

[93] Payabvash S, Tihan T, Cha S. Volumetric voxelwise apparent diffusion coefficient histogram analysis for differentiation of the fourth ventricular tumors. The Neuroradiology

Journal. 2018;**31**(6):554-564. DOI: 10.1177/1971400918800803

[94] Rodriguez Gutierrez D, Awwad A, Meijer L, Manita M, Jaspan T, et al. Metrics and textural features of MRI diffusion to improve classification of pediatric posterior fossa tumors. AJNR. American Journal of Neuroradiology. 2014;**35**(5):1009-1015. DOI: 10.3174/ajnr.A3784

[95] Rumboldt Z, Camacho DL, Lake D, Welsh CT, Castillo M. Apparent diffusion coefficients for differentiation of cerebellar tumors in children. AJNR. American Journal of Neuroradiology. 2006;**27**(6):1362-1369

[96] Schneider JF, Confort-Gouny S, Viola A, Le Fur Y, Viout P, Bennathan M, et al. Multiparametric differentiation of posterior fossa tumors in children using diffusion-weighted imaging and short echo-time 1H-MR spectroscopy. Journal of Magnetic Resonance Imaging. 2007;**26**(6):1390-1398. DOI: 10.1002/jmri.21185

[97] Wang W, Cheng J, Zhang Y, Wang C. Use of apparent diffusion coefficient histogram in differentiating between medulloblastoma and pilocytic astrocytoma in children. Medical Science Monitor. 2018;**24**:6107-6112. DOI: 10.12659/MSM.909136

[98] Dury RJ, Lourdusamy A, Macarthur DC, Peet AC, Auer DP, Grundy RG, et al. Meta-analysis of apparent diffusion coefficient in pediatric medulloblastoma, ependymoma, and pilocytic astrocytoma. Journal of Magnetic Resonance Imaging. 2022;**56**(1):147-157. DOI: 10.1002/jmri.28007

[99] Novak J, Zarinabad N, Rose H, Arvanitis T, MacPherson L, Pinkey B, et al. Classification of paediatric brain tumours by diffusion weighted imaging and machine learning. Scientific Reports. 2021;**11**(1):2987. DOI: 10.1038/s41598-021-82214-3

[100] Zhang M, Wong SW, Lummus S, Han M, Radmanesh A, Ahmadian SS, et al. Radiomic phenotypes distinguish atypical teratoid/rhabdoid tumors from medulloblastoma. AJNR. American Journal of Neuroradiology. 2021;**42**(9):1702-1708. DOI: 10.3174/ajnr.A7200

[101] Perreault S, Ramaswamy V, Achrol AS, Chao K, Liu TT, Shih D, et al. MRI surrogates for molecular subgroups of medulloblastoma. AJNR. American Journal of Neuroradiology. 2014;**35**(7):1263-1269. DOI: 10.3174/ajnr.A3990

[102] Łastowska M, Jurkiewicz E, Trubicka J, Daszkiewicz P, Drogosiewicz M, Malczyk K, et al. Contrast enhancement pattern predicts poor survival for patients with non-WNT/SHH medulloblastoma tumours. Journal of Neuro-Oncology. 2015;**123**(1):65-73. DOI: 10.1007/s11060-015-1779-0

[103] Patay Z, DeSain LA, Hwang SN, Coan A, Li Y, Ellison DW. MR imaging characteristics of wingless-type-subgroup pediatric medulloblastoma. AJNR. American Journal of Neuroradiology. 2015;**36**(12):2386-2393. DOI: 10.3174/ajnr.A4495

[104] Keil VC, Warmuth-Metz M, Reh C, Enkirch SJ, Reinert C, Beier D, et al. Imaging biomarkers for adult medulloblastomas: Genetic entities may be identified by their MR imaging radiophenotype. AJNR. American Journal of Neuroradiology. 2017;**38**(10):1892-1898. DOI: 10.3174/ajnr.A5313

[105] Zhao F, Li C, Zhou Q, Qu P, Wang B, Wang X, et al. Distinctive localization

and MRI features correlate of molecular subgroups in adult medulloblastoma. Journal of Neuro-Oncology. 2017;**135**(2):353-360. DOI: 10.1007/s11060-017-2581-y

[106] Mata-Mbemba D, Zapotocky M, Laughlin S, Taylor MD, Ramaswamy V, Raybaud C. MRI characteristics of primary tumors and metastatic lesions in molecular subgroups of pediatric medulloblastoma: A single-center study. AJNR. American Journal of Neuroradiology. 2018;**39**(5):949-955. DOI: 10.3174/ajnr.A5578

[107] Zapotocky M, Mata-Mbemba D, Sumerauer D, Liby P, Lassaletta A, Zamecnik J, et al. Differential patterns of metastatic dissemination across medulloblastoma subgroups. Journal of Neurosurgery. Pediatrics. 2018;**21**(2):145-152. DOI: 10.3171/2017.12.PEDS17264a

[108] Colafati GS, Voicu IP, Carducci C, Miele E, Carai A, Di Loreto S, et al. MRI features as a helpful tool to predict the molecular subgroups of medulloblastoma: State of the art. Therapeutic Advances in Neurological Disorders. 2018;**11**:1756286418775375. DOI: 10.1177/1756286418775375

[109] Zhang M, Wong SW, Wright JN, Wagner MW, Toescu S, Han M, et al. MRI radiogenomics of pediatric medulloblastoma: A multicenter study. Radiology. 2022;**304**(2):406-416. DOI: 10.1148/radiol.212137

[110] Ramaswamy V, Remke M, Bouffet E, Bailey S, Clifford SC, Doz F, et al. Risk stratification of childhood medulloblastoma in the molecular era: The current consensus. Acta Neuropathologica. 2016;**131**(6):821-831. DOI: 10.1007/s00401-016-1569-6

[111] Zeltzer PM, Boyett JM, Finlay JL, Albright AL, Rorke LB, Milstein JM, et al. Metastasis stage, adjuvant treatment, and residual tumor are prognostic factors for medulloblastoma in children: Conclusions from the Children's cancer group 921 randomized phase III study. Journal of Clinical Oncology. 1999;**17**(3):832-845. DOI: 10.1200/JCO.1999.17.3.832

[112] Robertson PL, Muraszko KM, Holmes EJ, Sposto R, Packer RJ, Gajjar A, et al. Incidence and severity of postoperative cerebellar mutism syndrome in children with medulloblastoma: A prospective study by the Children's oncology group. Journal of Neurosurgery. 2006;**105**(6 Suppl.):444-451. DOI: 10.3171/ped.2006.105.6.444

[113] Catsman-Berrevoets CE. Cerebellar mutism syndrome: Cause and rehabilitation. Current Opinion in Neurology. 2017;**30**(2):133-139. DOI: 10.1097/WCO.0000000000000426

[114] Pols SYCV, van Veelen MLC, Aarsen FK, Gonzalez Candel A, Catsman-Berrevoets CE. Risk factors for development of postoperative cerebellar mutism syndrome in children after medulloblastoma surgery. Journal of Neurosurgery. Pediatrics. 2017;**20**(1):35-41. DOI: 10.3171/2017.2.PEDS16605

[115] Torres CF, Rebsamen S, Silber JH, Sutton LN, Bilaniuk LT, Zimmerman RA, et al. Surveillance scanning of children with medulloblastoma. The New England Journal of Medicine. 1994;**330**(13):892-895. DOI: 10.1056/NEJM199403313301303

[116] Yalçin B, Büyükpamukçu M, Akalan N, Cila A, Kutluk MT, Akyüz C. Value of surveillance imaging in the management of medulloblastoma. Medical and Pediatric Oncology. 2002;**38**(2):91-97. DOI: 10.1002/mpo.1278

[117] Saunders DE, Hayward RD, Phipps KP, Chong WK, Wade AM. Surveillance neuroimaging of intracranial medulloblastoma in children: How effective, how often, and for how long? Journal of Neurosurgery. 2003;**99**(2):280-286. DOI: 10.3171/jns.2003.99.2.0280

[118] Taylor MD, Northcott PA, Korshunov A, Remke M, Cho YJ, Clifford SC, et al. Molecular subgroups of medulloblastoma: The current consensus. Acta Neuropathologica. 2012;**123**(4):465-472. DOI: 10.1007/s00401-011-0922-z

[119] Kool M, Korshunov A, Remke M, Jones DT, Schlanstein M, Northcott PA, et al. Molecular subgroups of medulloblastoma: An international meta-analysis of transcriptome, genetic aberrations, and clinical data of WNT, SHH, group 3, and group 4 medulloblastomas. Acta Neuropathologica. 2012;**123**(4):473-484. DOI: 10.1007/s00401-012-0958-8

[120] Ramaswamy V, Remke M, Bouffet E, Faria CC, Perreault S, Cho YJ, et al. Recurrence patterns across medulloblastoma subgroups: An integrated clinical and molecular analysis. The Lancet Oncology. 2013;**14**(12):1200-1207. DOI: 10.1016/S1470-2045(13)70449-2

[121] Bartels U, Shroff M, Sung L, Dag-Ellams U, Laperriere N, Rutka J, et al. Role of spinal MRI in the follow-up of children treated for medulloblastoma. Cancer. 2006;**107**(6):1340-1347. DOI: 10.1002/cncr.22129

[122] Morana G, Alves CA, Tortora D, Severino M, Nozza P, Cama A, et al. Added value of diffusion weighted imaging in pediatric central nervous system embryonal tumors surveillance. Oncotarget. 2017;**8**(36):60401-60413. DOI: 10.18632/oncotarget.19553

[123] Aboian MS, Kline CN, Li Y, Solomon DA, Felton E, Banerjee A, et al. Early detection of recurrent medulloblastoma: The critical role of diffusion-weighted imaging. Neurooncology Practice. 2018;**5**(4):234-240. DOI: 10.1093/nop/npx036

[124] Stavinoha PL, Askins MA, Powell SK, Pillay Smiley N, Robert RS. Neurocognitiveandpsychosocialoutcomes in pediatric brain tumor survivors. Bioengineering (Basel). 2018;**5**(3):73. DOI: 10.3390/bioengineering5030073

[125] Tonning Olsson I, Perrin S, Lundgren J, Hjorth L, Johanson A. Long-term cognitive sequelae after pediatric brain tumor related to medical risk factors, age, and sex. Pediatric Neurology. 2014;**51**(4):515-521. DOI: 10.1016/j.pediatrneurol.2014.06.011

[126] Józefacka NM, Machnikowska-Sokołowska MD, Kołek MF, Gruszczyńska KJ, Musioł K. Cognitive performance of medulloblastoma tumour survivors related to the area of cerebellum damage. Reports of Practical Oncology and Radiotherapy. 2022;**27**(6):1037-1044. DOI: 10.5603/RPOR.a2022.0105